COVID-19 Meeting the Challenge

AF599041

Living in Lockdown

Samantha Kohn

CRABTREE
PUBLISHING COMPANY
WWW.CRABTREEBOOKS.COM

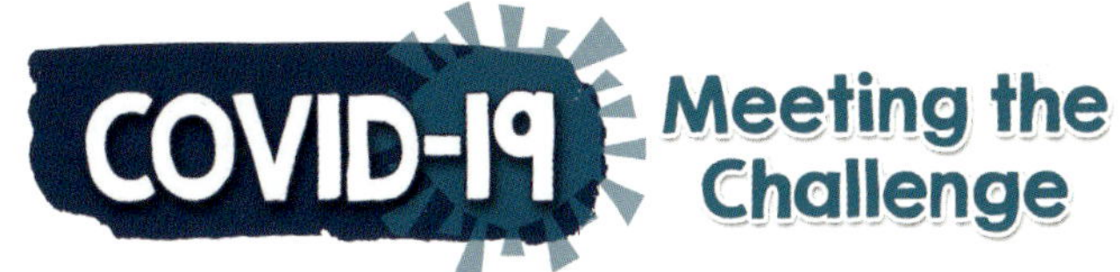

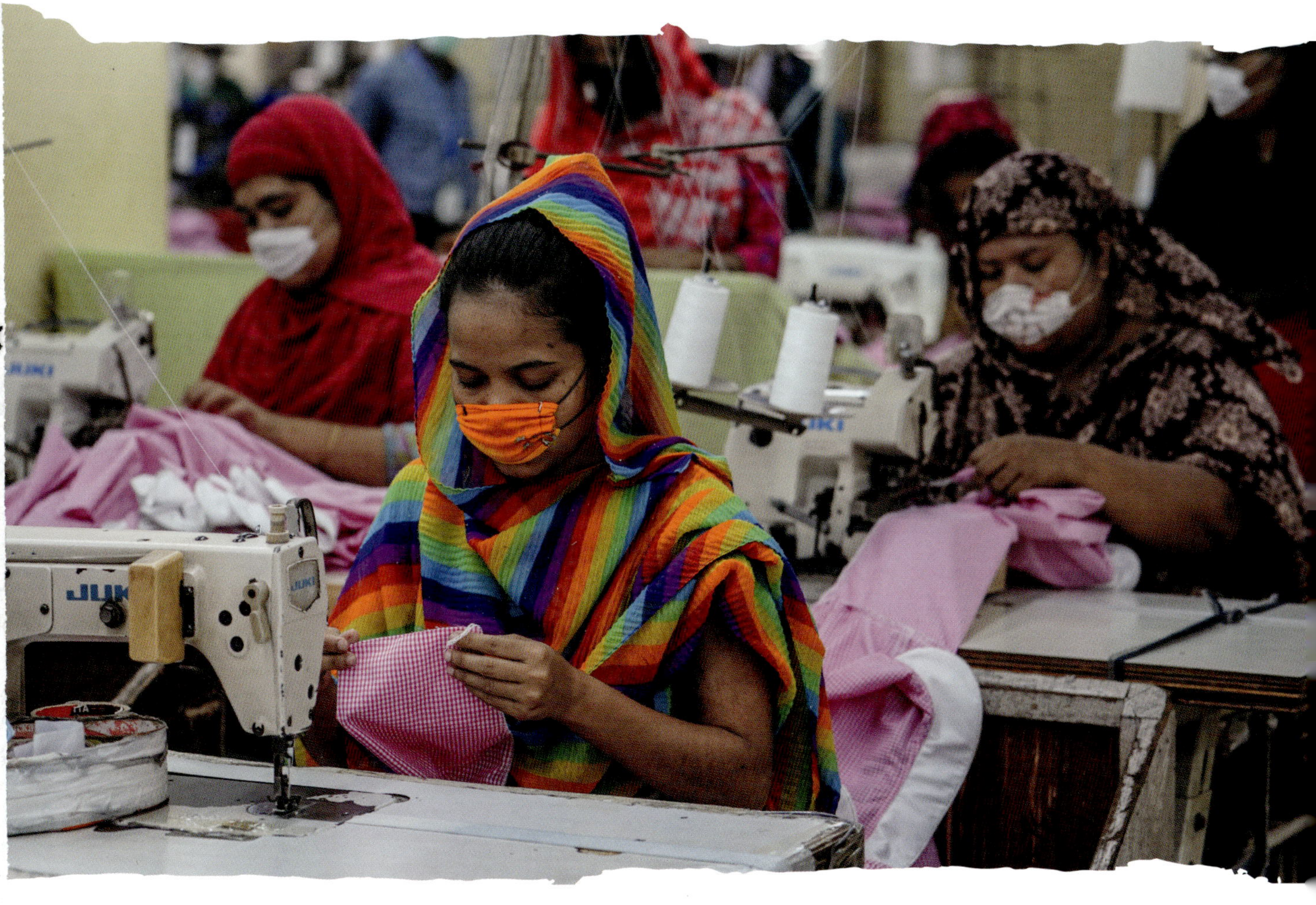

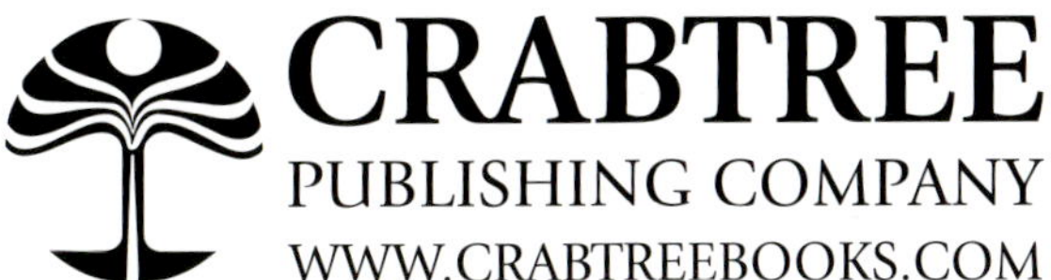

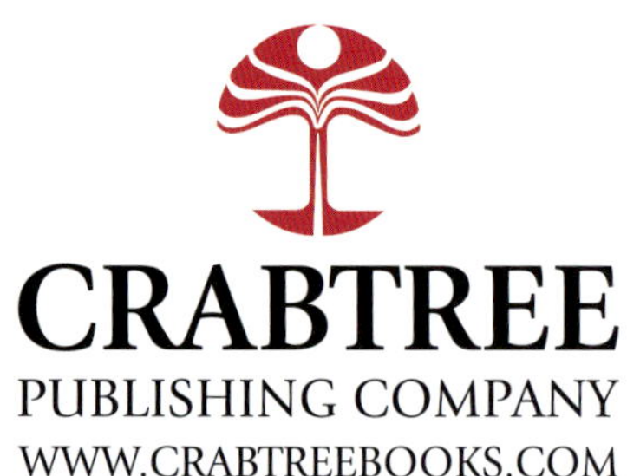

Author:
Samantha Kohn

Series research and development:
Janine Deschenes and Ellen Rodger

Editorial director:
Kathy Middleton

Editors:
Janine Deschenes and Ellen Rodger

Proofreader:
Wendy Scavuzzo

Graphic design:
Samara Parent

Image research:
Samara Parent

Print coordinator:
Katherine Berti

Images:
Alamy
Maridav: p. 3
Jayne Russell: p. 12-13
Newscom: p. 14-15
REUTERS: p. 32

Ashlee Ellison Photography: p. 34

The Canadian Press
Darryl Dyck: p. 21

Shutterstock
Zabed Hasnain Chowdhury: title page
Mark Brandon: p. 4-5 (top)
Dave Hewison Photography: p. 6
YES Market Media: p. 7
Sara Sette: p. 13
Colin Giesbrecht: p. 15
EQRoy: p. 16
Vera Eremova: p. 17
Vladirina32: p. 18-19
Chris Allan: p. 20
Tada Images: p. 22-23
nevada.claire: p. 24-25
blvdone: p. 26
Naresh777: p. 27 (bottom right)
JessicaGirvan: p. 30
Kyle Oster: p. 31 (top)
Exposure Visuals: p. 34-35
John Doukas: p. 36
ChameleonsEye: p. 37
Vipavlenkoff: p. 38
Matt Gush: p. 38-39
Travers Lewis: p. 40 (top)
kandl stock: p. 40 (bottom)
Alexandros Michailidis: p. 41
Elena Fontana Photography: p. 42
RightFramePhotoVideo: p. 45

Wikimedia Commons
Scotted400: p. 11

All other images by Shutterstock

Library and Archives Canada Cataloguing in Publication

Title: Living in lockdown / Samantha Kohn.
Names: Kohn, Samantha, author.
Description: Series statement: COVID-19: meeting the challenge | Includes bibliographical references and index.
Identifiers: Canadiana (print) 20210248742 | Canadiana (ebook) 20210248769 | ISBN 9781427156082 (hardcover) | ISBN 9781427156105 (softcover) | ISBN 9781427156129 (HTML) | ISBN 9781427156440 (EPUB)
Subjects: LCSH: COVID-19 Pandemic, 2020—Safety measures—Juvenile literature. | LCSH: COVID-19 Pandemic, 2020—Social aspects—Juvenile literature. | LCSH: COVID-19 (Disease)—Safety measures—Juvenile literature. | LCSH: COVID-19 (Disease)—Social aspects—Juvenile literature. | LCSH: Public health—Safety measures—Juvenile literature. | LCSH: Public health—Social aspects—Juvenile literature.
Classification: LCC RA644.C67 K67 2022 | DDC j614.5/92414—dc23

Library of Congress Cataloging-in-Publication Data

Names: Kohn, Samantha, author.
Title: Living in lockdown / Samantha Kohn.
Description: New York, NY : Crabtree Publishing Company, [2022] | Series: COVID-19: meeting the challenge | Includes index.
Identifiers: LCCN 2021027942 (print) | LCCN 2021027943 (ebook) | ISBN 9781427156082 (hardcover) | ISBN 9781427156105 (paperback) | ISBN 9781427156129 (ebook) | ISBN 9781427156440 (epub)
Subjects: LCSH: Health planning--Decision making--Juvenile literature. | Medical policy--Decision making--Juvenile literature. | COVID-19 (Disease)--Social aspects--Juvenile literature. | COVID-19 (Disease)--Economic aspects--Juvenile literature. | Epidemics--Juvenile literature.
Classification: LCC RA393 .K64 2022 (print) | LCC RA393 (ebook) | DDC 614.5/92414--dc23
LC record available at https://lccn.loc.gov/2021027942
LC ebook record available at https://lccn.loc.gov/2021027943

Crabtree Publishing Company

www.crabtreebooks.com 1-800-387-7650

In Canada: We acknowledge the financial support of the Government of Canada through the Canada Book Fund for our publishing activities.

Published in Canada
Crabtree Publishing
616 Welland Ave.
St. Catharines, Ontario
L2M 5V6

Published in the United States
Crabtree Publishing
347 Fifth Ave
Suite 1402-145
New York, NY 10016

Printed in the U.S.A./092021/CG20210616

CONTENTS

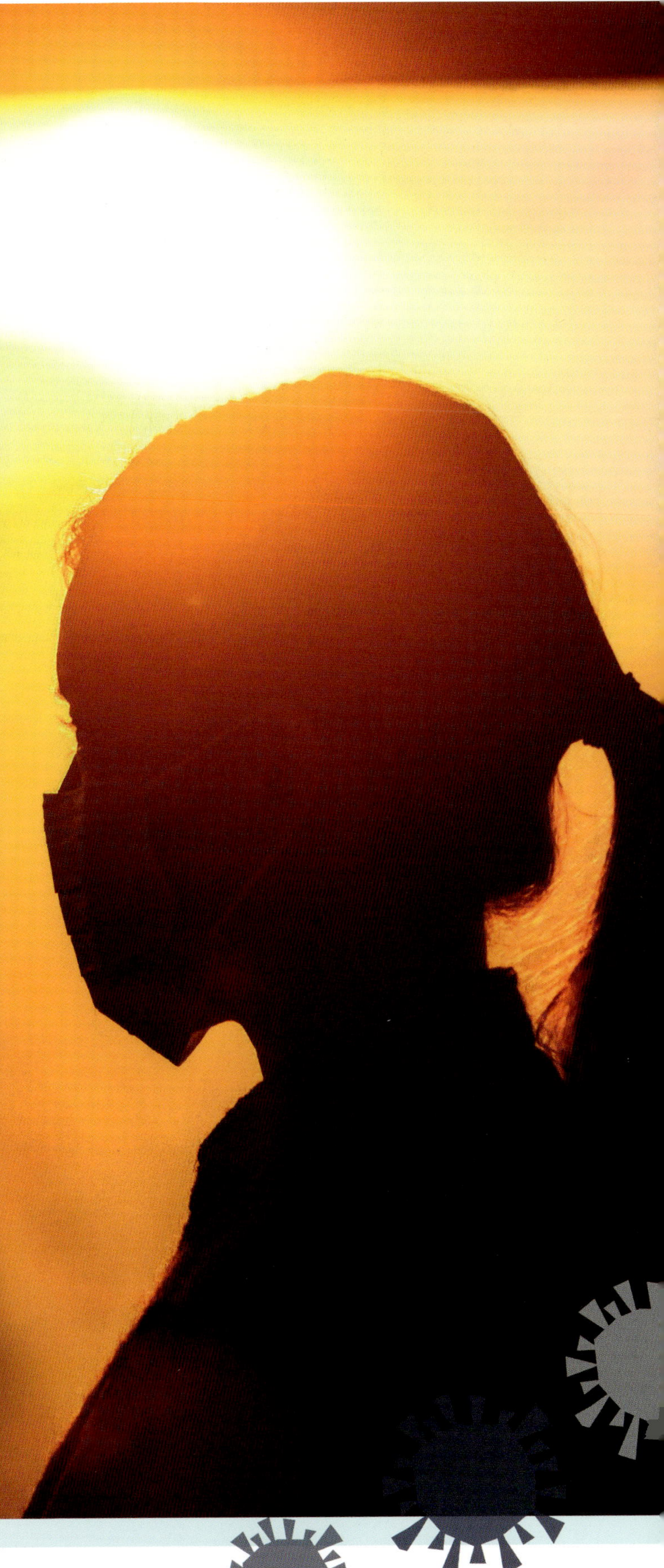

Introduction

It was late at night on January 25, 2020, and Zhi Ruo Yong couldn't sleep. She wasn't worried about being tired the next morning, though. She knew she wouldn't have to wake up for school, anyway.

Zhi lived in Wuhan, China, a city of 11 million people. Her city had been in **lockdown** for two days. A mysterious virus was filling the city's hospitals with very sick patients. Residents of Wuhan were not allowed to leave the city. All buses, trains, flights, ferries, and major highways had been shut down. People were only allowed to leave their homes to shop for food. By mid-February 2020, all **non-essential** businesses in the province of Hubei were closed, and people were no longer allowed to leave their homes. All supplies were delivered, and delivery drivers became lifesaving heroes.

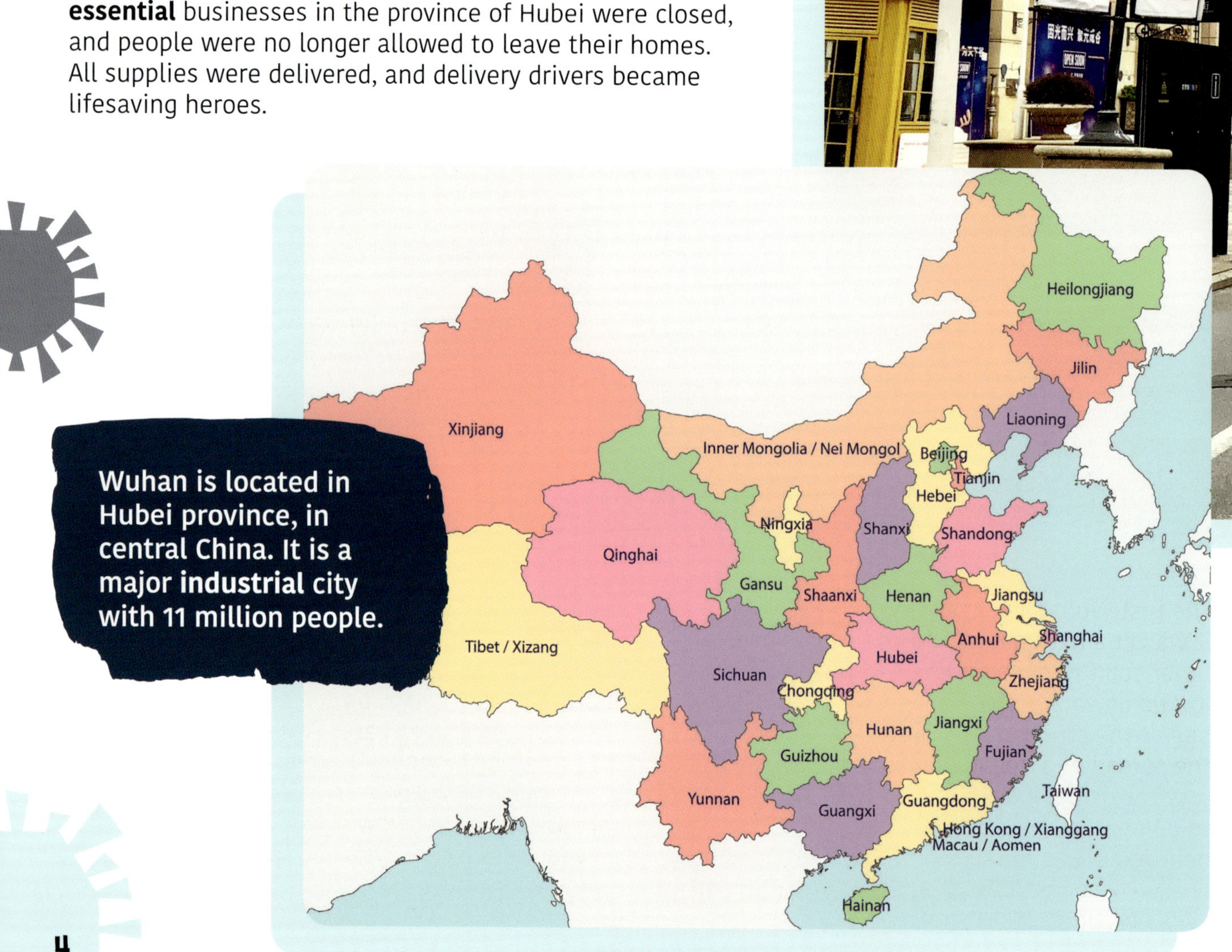

Wuhan is located in Hubei province, in central China. It is a major industrial city with 11 million people.

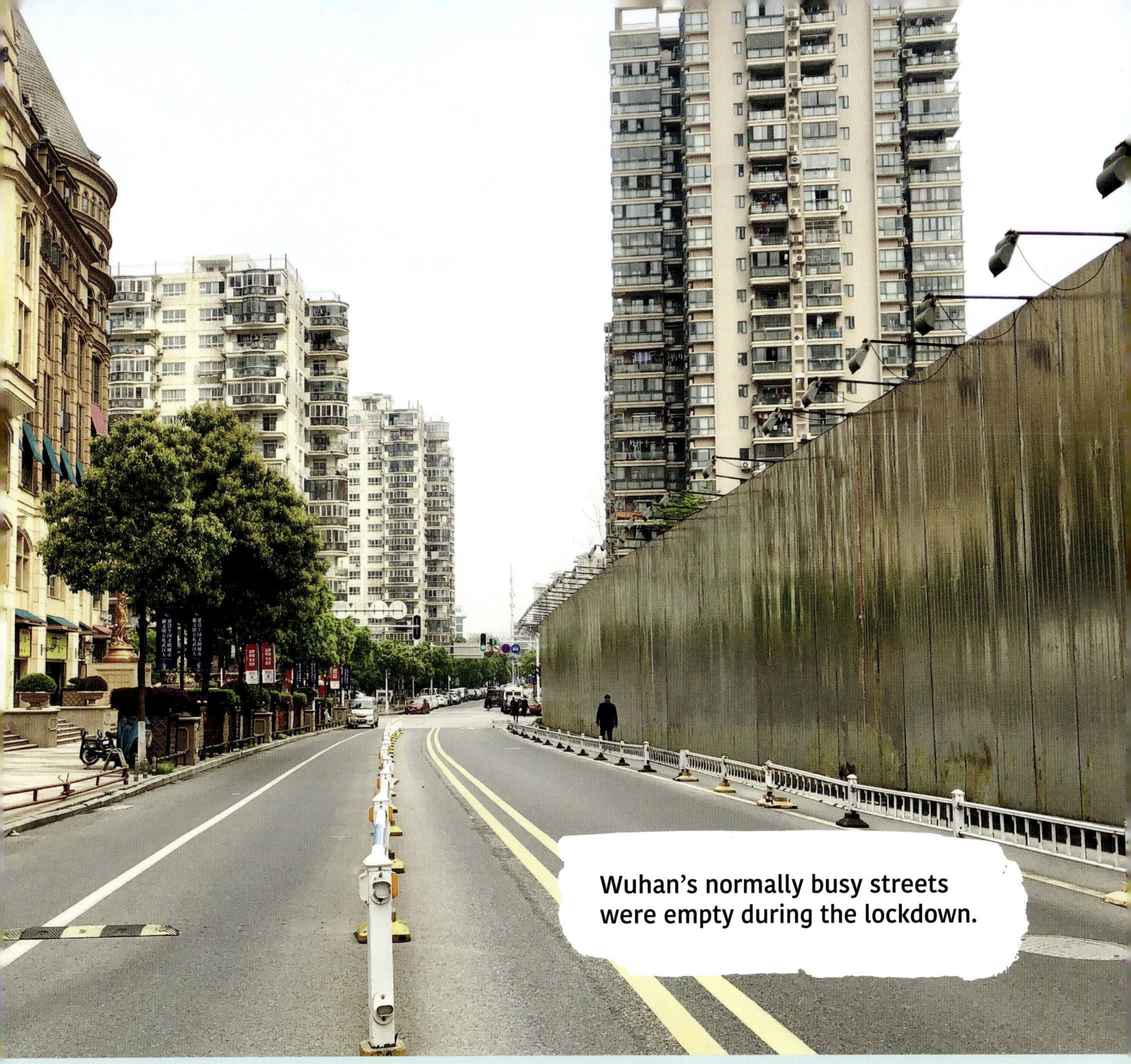

Wuhan's normally busy streets were empty during the lockdown.

The first Wuhan lockdown lasted 76 days. While it wasn't a national lockdown like the ones in other countries, the number of people who were locked down and the tight restrictions made it one of the strictest. The lockdown aimed to slow the spread of a novel, or new, **coronavirus** that was causing the disease COVID-19. It was hard to pinpoint where the virus began, but scientists believed it was passed from animals to humans. It quickly spread, causing many people to get very sick, and causing some to die.

Within weeks, North American and European governments watched in anticipation as hospitals filled with patients in other countries. Lockdowns seemed to be the only way of slowing the spread of the disease. Everyone knew that it couldn't be stopped. However, if people were kept home and away from one another, the spread could slow. Slowing the spread would prevent health care systems from having too many sick people all at once.

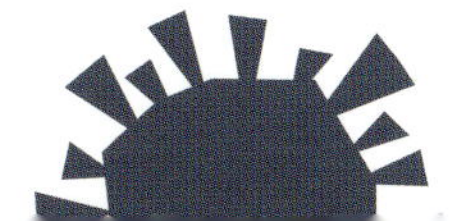

Chapter 1

Lockdowns Begin

Nearly every country in the world had some form of lockdown in 2020. Some governments extended lockdowns well into 2021. Every lockdown was different. Some were longer and stricter than others.

New Normals

In some places, people were only allowed to leave their homes for essential reasons, such as shopping for food or going to a doctor's appointment. In other places, people were not allowed to leave their homes at all. Some countries had strict, national lockdowns in which every person faced the same restrictions no matter where they lived. Other countries only put certain cities, states, or provinces under lockdown. Some countries, such as Australia, locked down just one or two cities when the number of positive COVID-19 cases increased. The country decided in May 2021 to ban foreign travel until 2022. A few countries had no lockdowns at all—at least in the beginning of the **pandemic**.

By early April, 2020, 3.9 billion people around the world were under some form of lockdown. That's about half of the world's population!

An important message from the Victorian Government
STAGE 3 RESTRICTIONS ARE NOW IN PLACE. GO HOME.
Find out more at coronavirus.vic.gov.au
VICTORIA
Managing this together
QMS

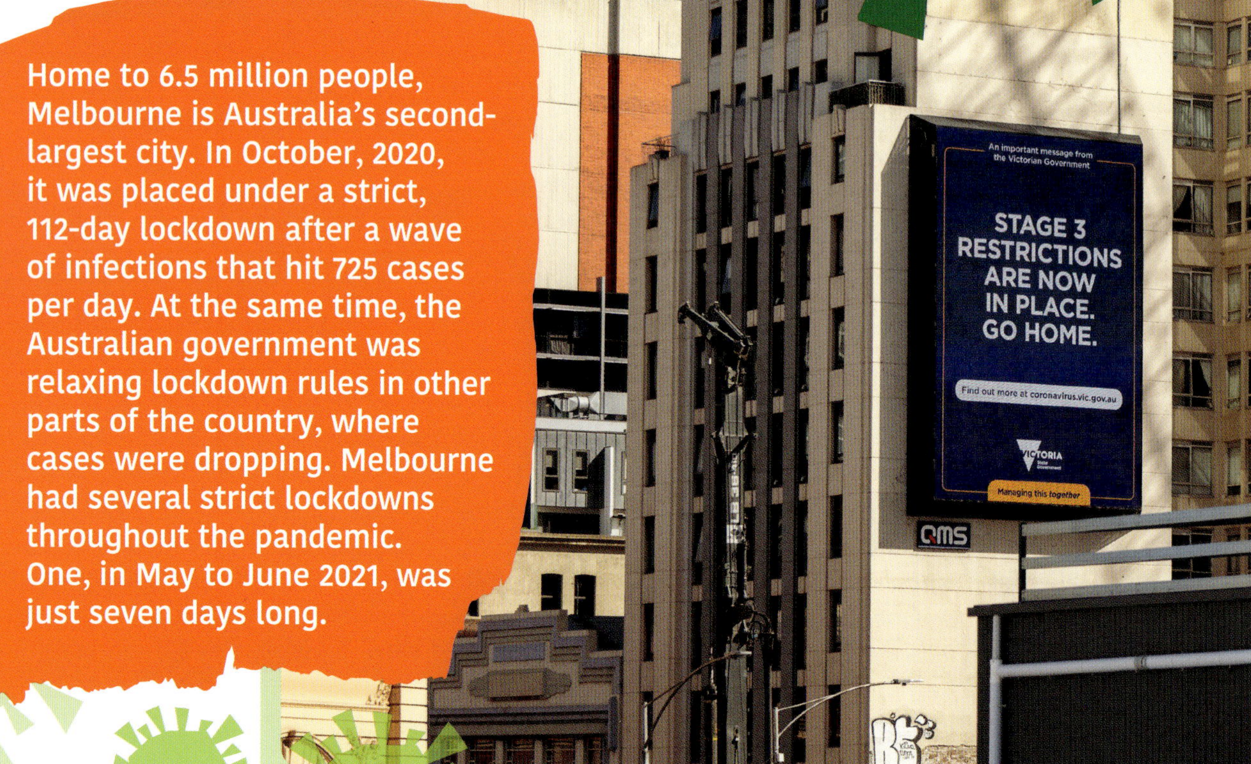

Home to 6.5 million people, Melbourne is Australia's second-largest city. In October, 2020, it was placed under a strict, 112-day lockdown after a wave of infections that hit 725 cases per day. At the same time, the Australian government was relaxing lockdown rules in other parts of the country, where cases were dropping. Melbourne had several strict lockdowns throughout the pandemic. One, in May to June 2021, was just seven days long.

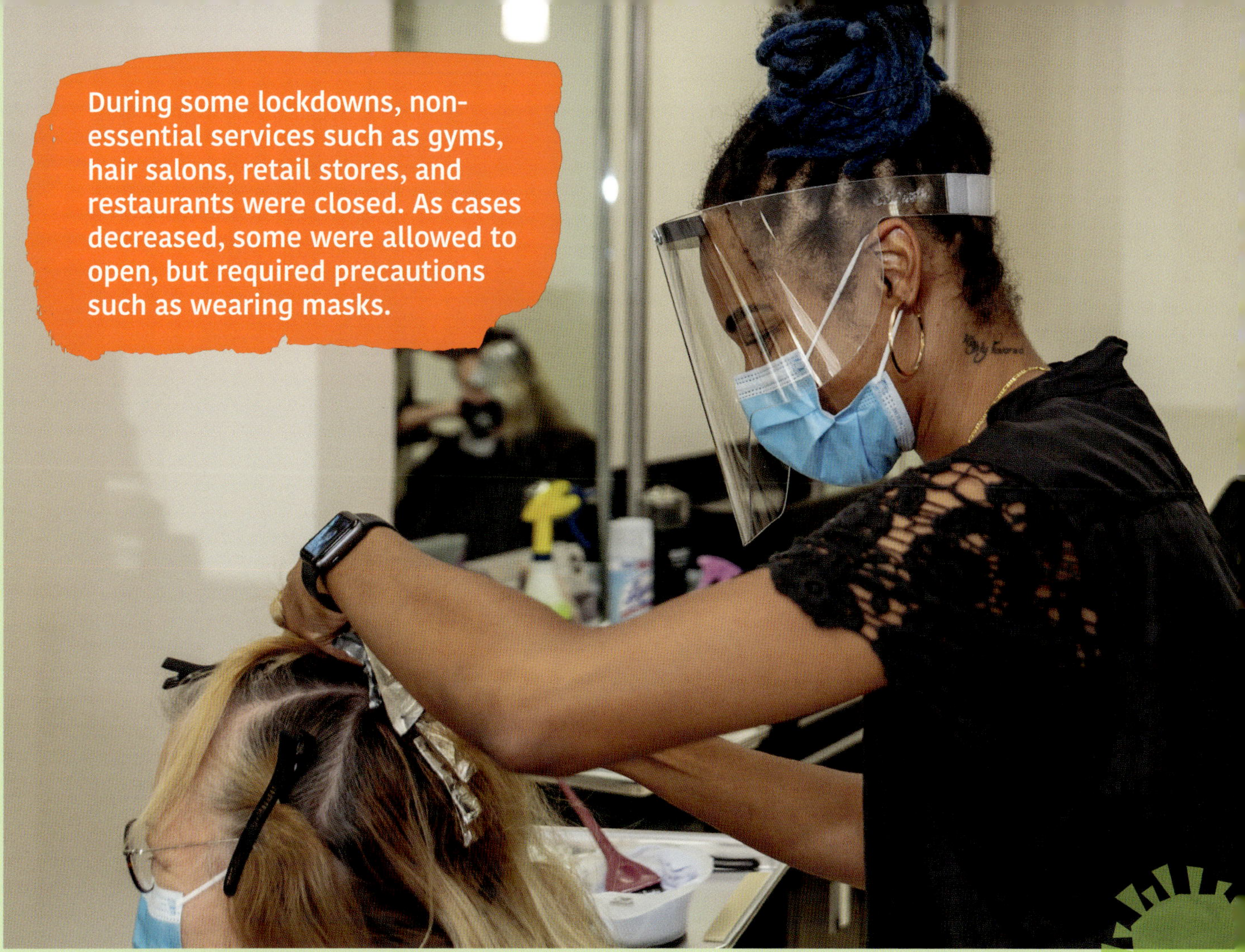

During some lockdowns, non-essential services such as gyms, hair salons, retail stores, and restaurants were closed. As cases decreased, some were allowed to open, but required precautions such as wearing masks.

Rules and Restrictions

Every lockdown was different. In the South American country of Colombia, people were only allowed to leave their homes on certain days. Those days were determined by the number on their **national ID cards**. In the European country of Serbia, dog owners were only allowed to walk their dogs from 8 to 9 p.m. Eventually, walking dogs was banned entirely as the number of infections continued to rise. The Serbian government struggled to keep the virus under control, and strict rules such as **curfews** were imposed. In Ireland, people were only allowed to leave their homes for food or exercise. They were also not allowed to be more than 3.1 miles (5 km) away from their homes. But while all lockdowns were different, there were a few restrictions that were part of nearly all of them.

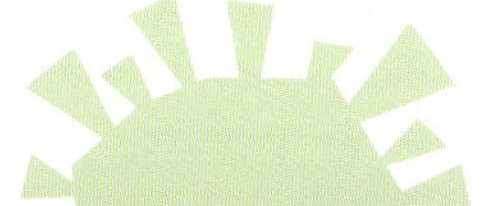

Lockdown Basics

Since the virus that caused COVID-19 spread so easily, **public health** agencies advised that everyone needed to follow some simple measures to prevent infections. These included wearing face masks, frequent handwashing, keeping 6 feet (2 m) away from others, and not gathering with people from other households. The idea was to slow the numbers of sick people who needed hospital care. Lockdowns restricted movement, which helped keep people from coming in contact with others and spreading the virus. Mandatory mask wearing in public spaces was a big part of many lockdown regulations. Governments also limited the size of public gatherings. These varied according to the severity of the lockdown. In some cases, gatherings were limited to no more than 5 to 10 people.

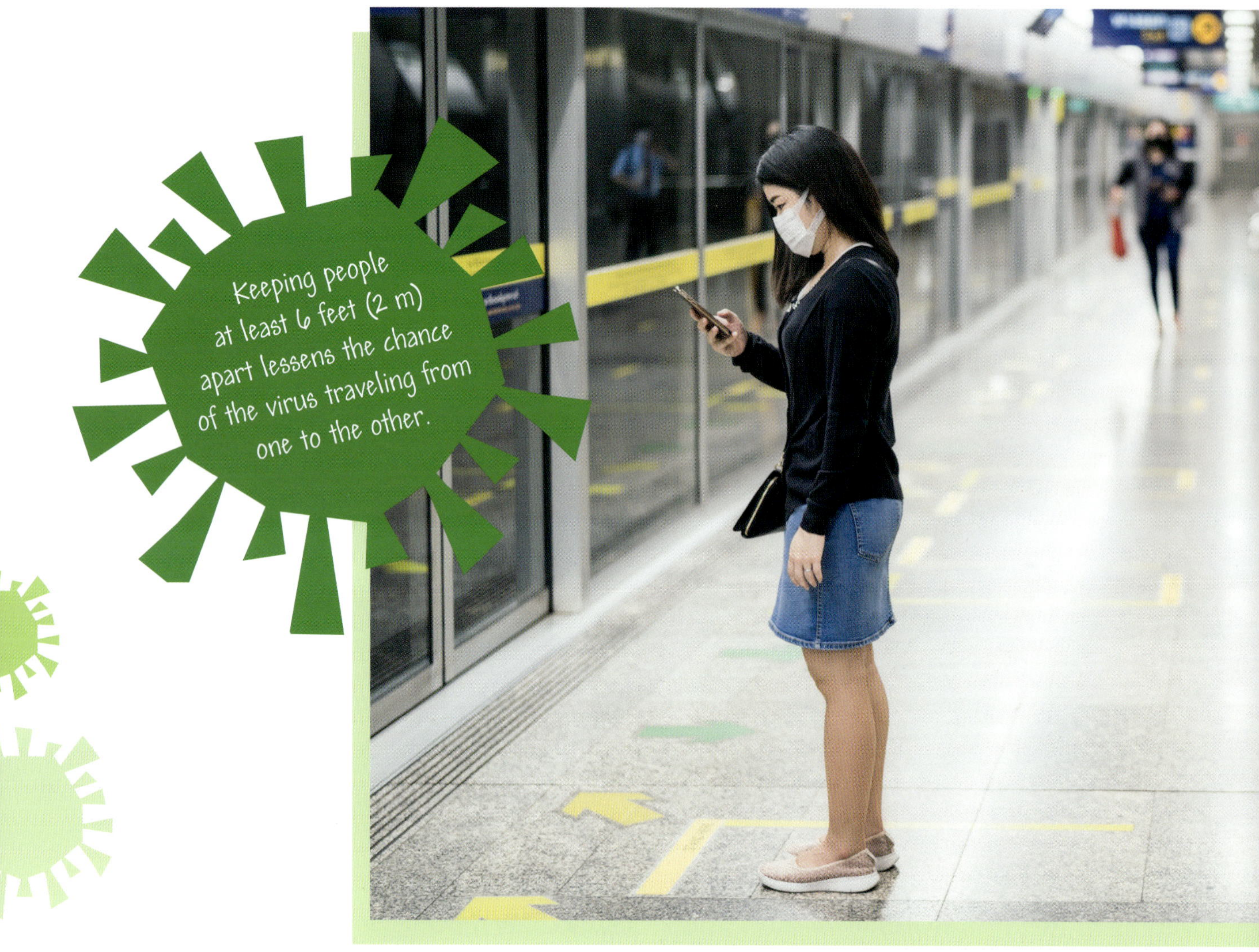

Keeping people at least 6 feet (2 m) apart lessens the chance of the virus traveling from one to the other.

How Viruses Spread

How do lockdowns prevent people from getting sick? The answer to that lies in the science of how viruses spread. Viruses are tiny organisms, or living things, that can infect other living things. They need a **host** to survive. Once they find that host, the virus causes an infection. The host can spread the virus to other living things.

A New Virus

COVID-19 is a disease caused by the SARS-CoV-2 virus. It is a new coronavirus that was first detected in Wuhan, China, in December 2019. It is believed to have spread from an animal source to humans. Coronaviruses can infect your nose, sinuses, or upper throat. They are named for the spikes that resemble a crown, or corona, that can only be seen through powerful microscopes. Because it is novel, or new to humans, SARS-CoV-2 caused a disease to which humans were not **immune**.

COVID-19 spreads by **droplets**. That means a person has to be in contact with someone who already has the virus to catch the disease. When the sick person speaks, sings, coughs, sneezes, or breathes, they release little droplets into the air. There is COVID-19 in those droplets. The droplets can travel several feet or meters. If someone nearby inhales those droplets, or the droplets get into the healthy person's eyes, nose, or mouth, the virus could infect that person.

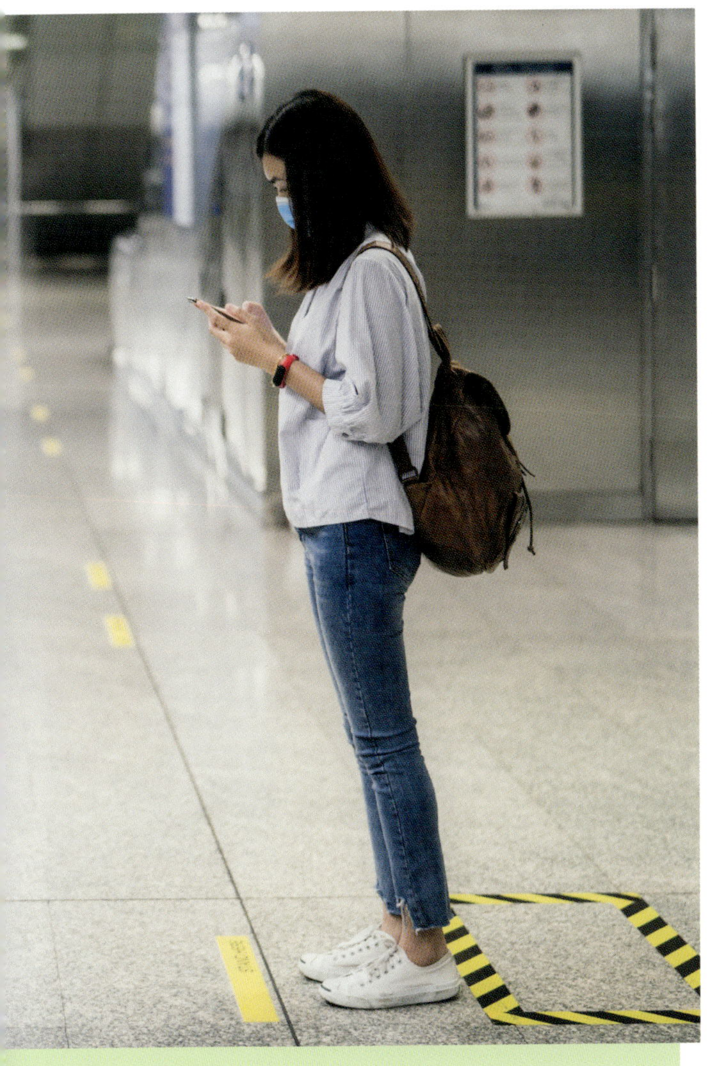

The Health Care System

There are only so many beds in a hospital. There are only so many nurses and doctors to take care of patients. With COVID-19's rapid spread, the fear was that there wouldn't be enough hospital beds or health care workers to care for sick people. For that reason, medical professionals encouraged lockdowns. They wanted to help make sure that when people got sick, health care systems would be able to handle all of the patients and give them proper care.

Flattening the Curve

Slowing down the spread of the virus was called "flattening the curve." In the study of diseases, the number of new cases is often placed on a graph that also shows the ability of a health care system to care for the people needing hospitalization. The curve is the **projected** number of new cases that are expected over a period of time. When a disease spreads, there is a spike in the curve of new infections. Sometimes, that spike rises above the line that shows how many people a health care system can care for. A flatter curve means fewer virus **transmissions** over a longer period, so hospitals can care for everyone.

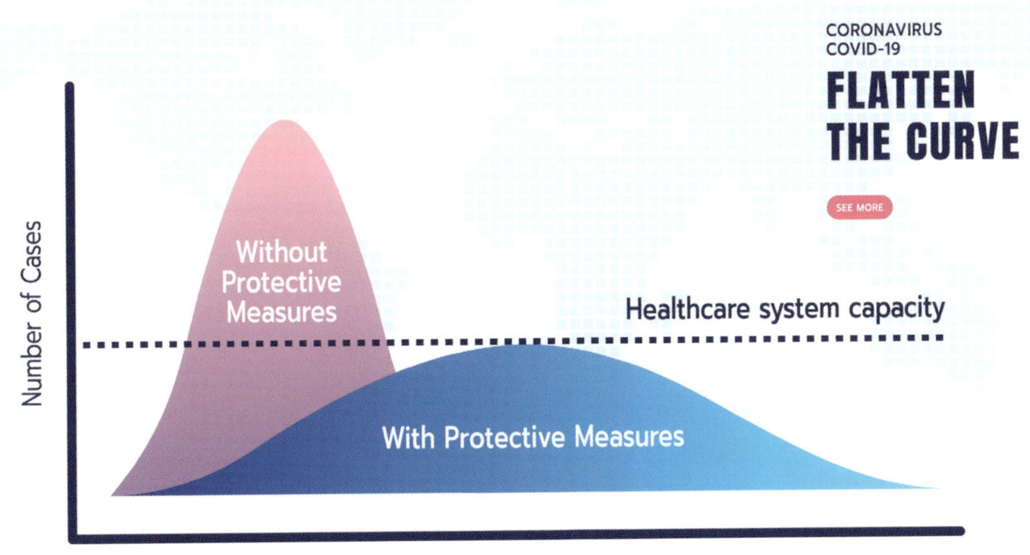

Measuring Contagiousness

A common way of measuring the **contagiousness** of a virus is by looking at its "R0" number. R0, pronounced "R naught," is the average number of people who will contract a disease from one infected person. For example, if a disease has an R0 of 3, a person who has the disease will spread it to an average of 3 other people. Then each of those people will spread it to 3 others, and so on. Why is the R0 important? If no measures were taken to reduce the spread of COVID-19, the virus would have an R0 of 5.7. That means COVID-19 is a very contagious disease. Without preventative measures such as lockdowns, it spread very quickly.

Studying Outbreaks

The R0 is one of the many tools epidemiologists, or disease scientists, use to study disease outbreaks. During the COVID-19 pandemic, they used it to determine when and where an outbreak was growing. Since the disease replicates, or copies, itself quickly, knowing how it would spread in an area over time was vital to ensuring health care services could cope with what was to come.

R0 numbers were determined by laboratory testing for positive cases.

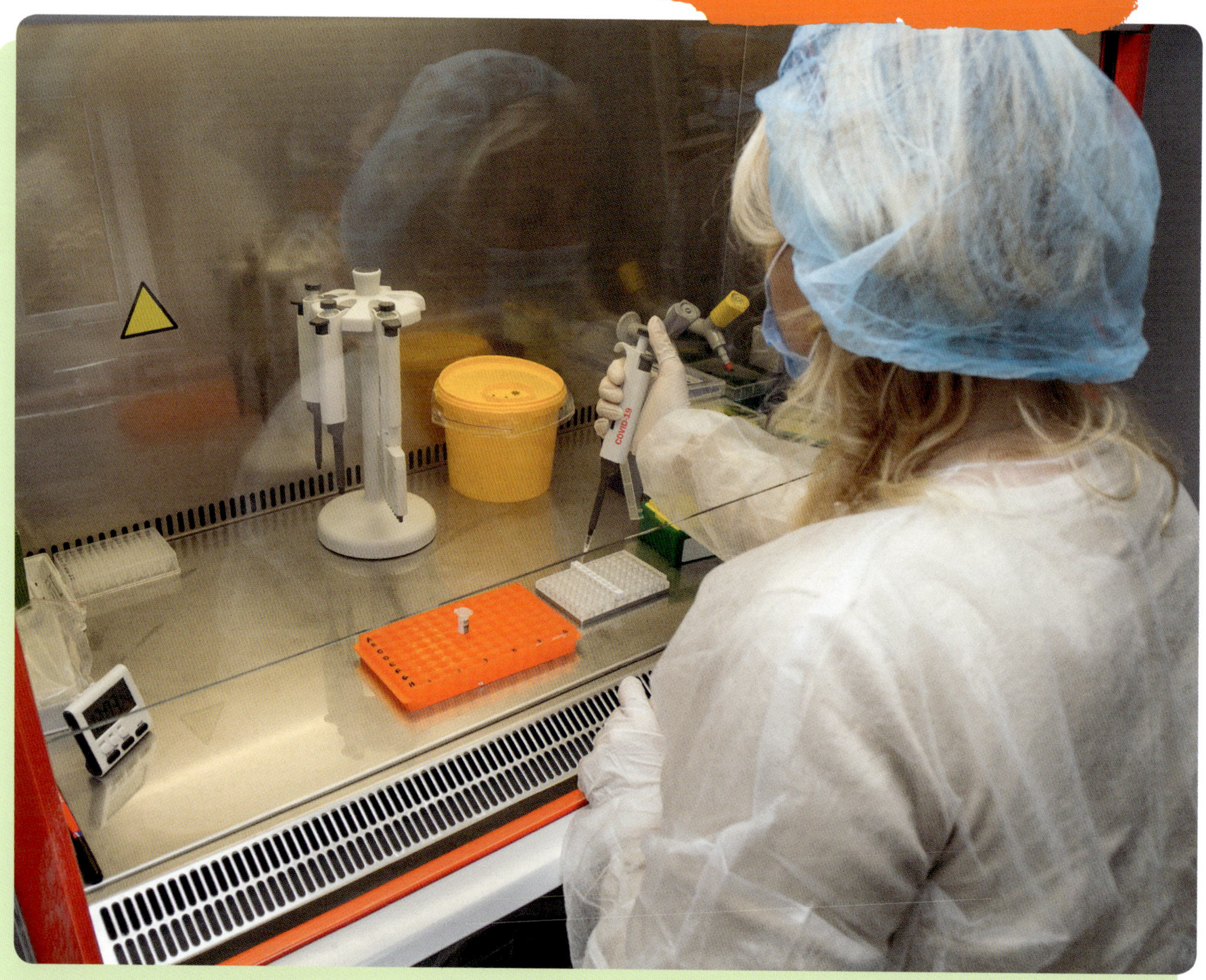

PANDEMIC WHO'S WHO

Zhang Yongzhen

Virologist Zhang Yongzhen works at the Shanghai Public Health Clinical Center in Shanghai, China. On January 3, 2020, his laboratory received a sample of the new coronavirus. His task was to study the virus and **sequence** it. Sequencing determines the structure of a virus, or how it is made up. This information would be used to understand the virus, develop tests for it, and create treatments and **vaccines**. Zhang's lab worked 40 hours straight to determine that the new virus was related to Severe Acute Respiratory Syndrome (SARS). SARS was a coronavirus that caused a deadly outbreak in 2003. The Chinese government had forbidden Chinese scientists from publishing information about the new virus. Zhang said he didn't know about this, however, and sent his data to the National Center for Biotechnology Information (NCBI) in the United States. He also submitted a paper to a journal for other scientists to read. He allowed a fellow scientist in Australia to release the information on the virus. Zhang had sequenced thousands of viruses in his career, but sequencing the coronavirus that causes COVID-19 was his fastest work. It allowed scientists all over the world to begin research on life-saving treatments and vaccines.

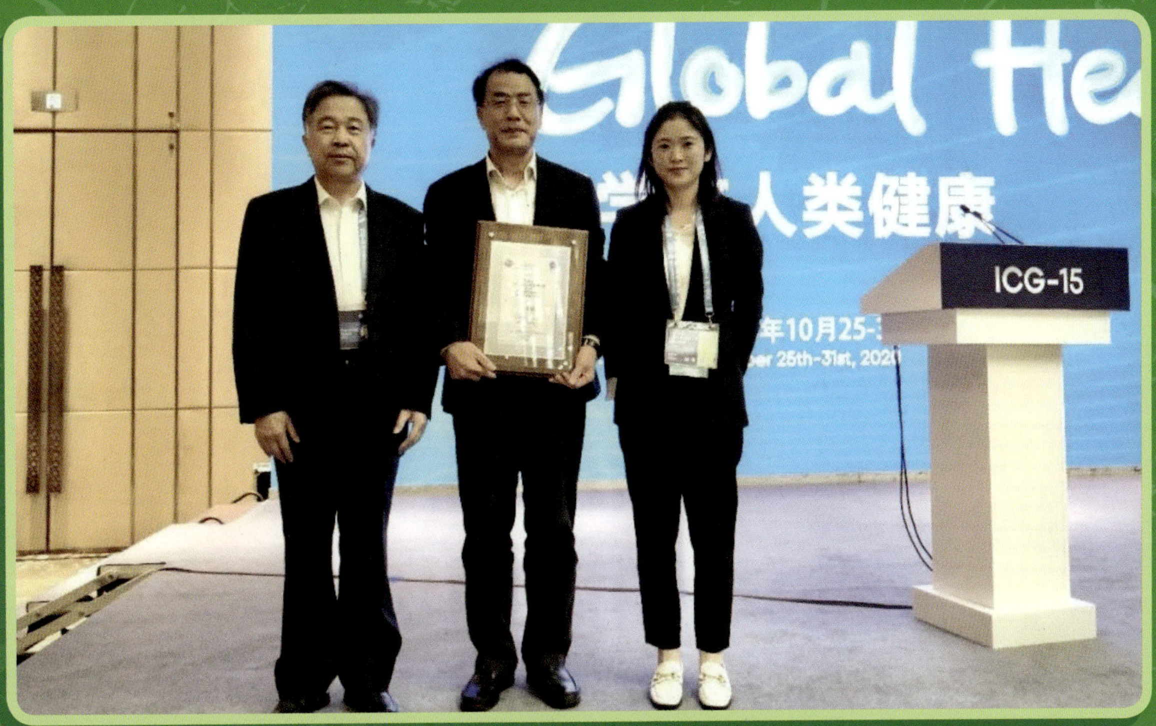

Zhang visited Wuhan to get information from doctors on how the virus affected people. He accepted an award for data sharing in 2020.

Lockdowns Begin

The first COVID-19 lockdowns were in China and Italy. Once the Chinese government realized how contagious and deadly the virus was, it acted to contain it. On January 18, 2020, the Chinese government sent disease experts to Wuhan. They studied what was then thought to be a local outbreak. In a Chinese television interview, epidemiologist Li Lanjuan called for an immediate lockdown. She felt that if the infection was allowed to continue, it would spread widely, kill many, and harm the Chinese **economy**. Li was respected for her work during earlier disease outbreaks, so the Chinese government acted on the advice of scientists. It shut down Wuhan, a city of 11 million, for months. Lockdowns followed in nearby cities in the same province of Hubei. That was the first time a city and province so large had been locked down to stop a disease.

By April 2020, more than 3.9 million people in 90 countries were under some form of lockdown. That was about half the world's population. Each lockdown differed, as each country used different COVID-19 coping strategies.

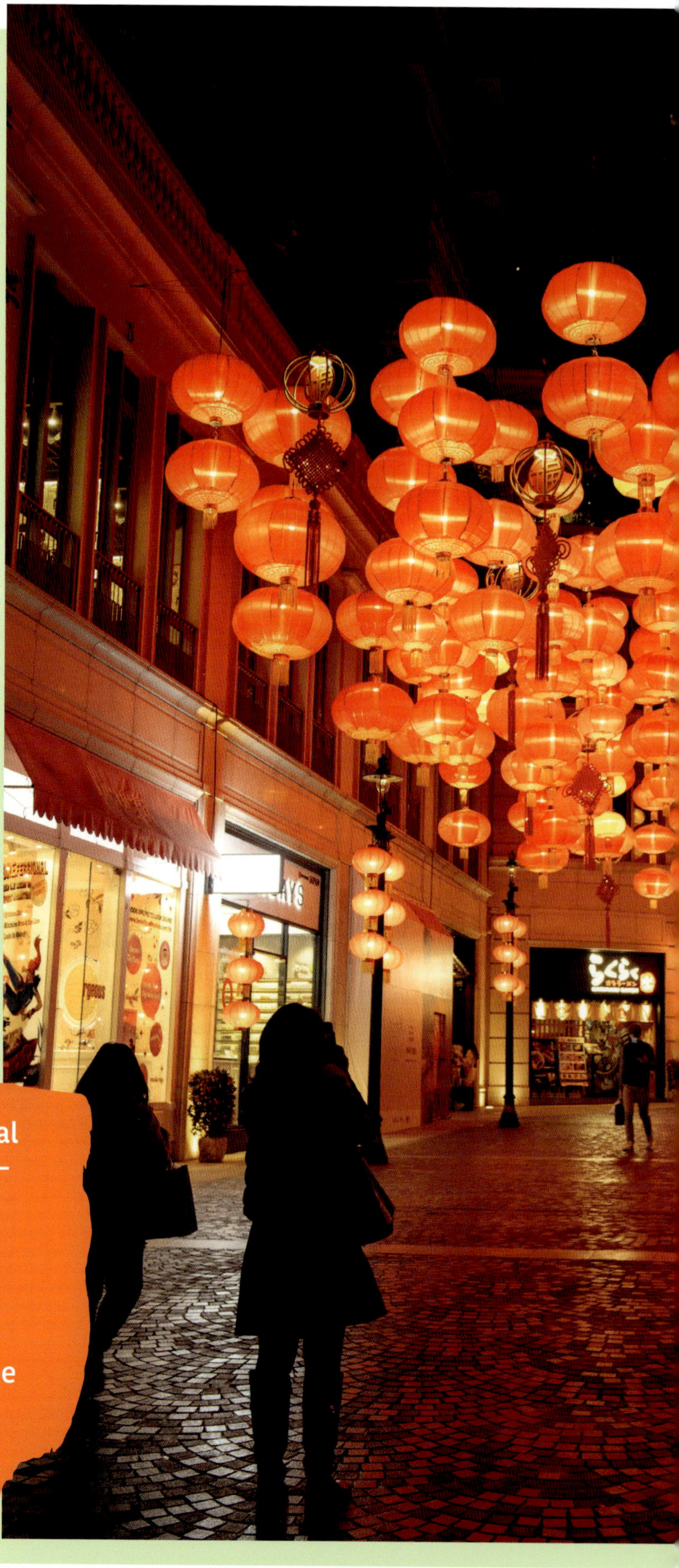

With the country's biggest national holiday—Chinese Lunar New Year—approaching on January 25, 2020, China wanted to make sure the virus didn't spread farther. China imposed a travel ban throughout the country on January 23. Lunar New Year is the biggest travel time in the country. Usually, millions of people travel to visit family in other cities.

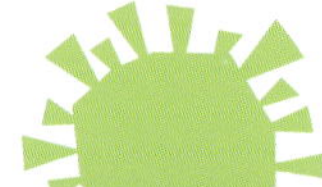

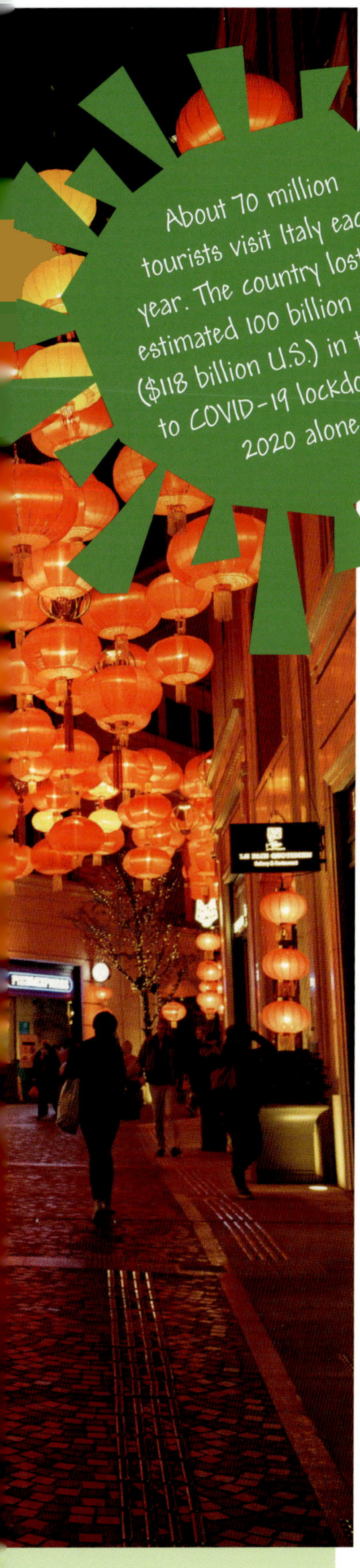

About 70 million tourists visit Italy each year. The country lost an estimated 100 billion euros ($118 billion U.S.) in tourism to COVID-19 lockdowns in 2020 alone.

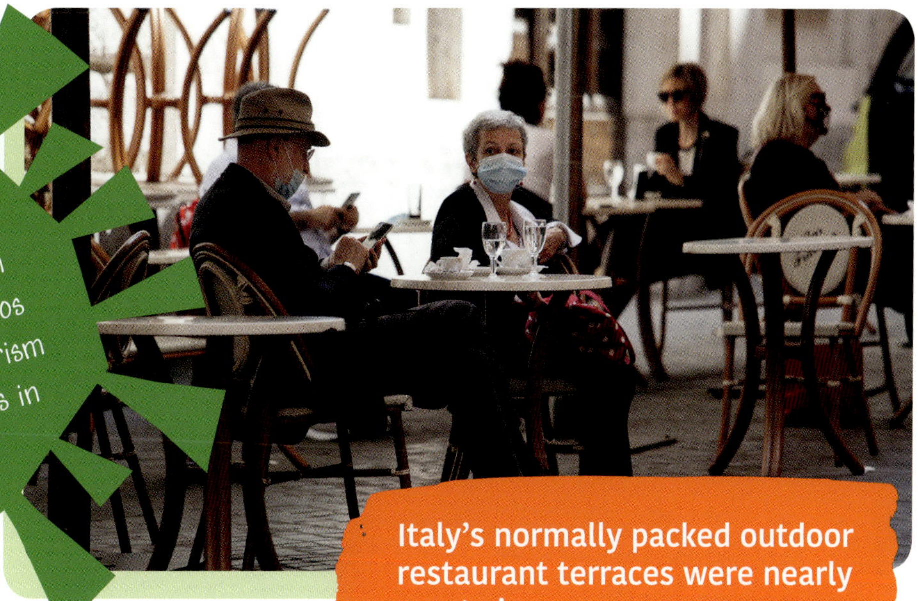

Italy's normally packed outdoor restaurant terraces were nearly empty in summer 2020.

Italy in Lockdown

On January 31, 2020, two cases of COVID-19 were confirmed in Italy's capital city of Rome. The Italian government immediately prevented all flights from Wuhan, China, from landing in Italy. However, the virus was already spreading through the population. With no social distancing measures in place and citizens still attending major events such as soccer matches and concerts, the virus spread quickly across northern Italy. In fact, one Italian soccer match on February 19, 2020, was later labeled a super spreader event. Super spreader events are mass gatherings in which people who had the virus attended and spread it unknowingly to others. The Italian match, played in Milan, is believed to have spread the virus to 40,000 people. Over the next two weeks, small towns and eventually provinces were placed under lockdown across the northern part of the country. Travel was also restricted between regions. The lockdown was then extended to the whole country on March 9, 2020. All 60 million people living in Italy were told to stay home.

Easing Lockdowns

Lockdown restrictions eased by May and June 2020 but, in October, the country was hit by a second wave of the virus. Restrictions were again put into place. By December 2020, the first COVID-19 vaccines were introduced. Vaccinations helped the country slowly open up again in early summer 2021. Like many European countries, Italy introduced a system in summer 2021 to allow tourists to visit from countries with similar vaccination rates.

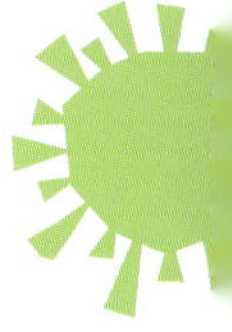

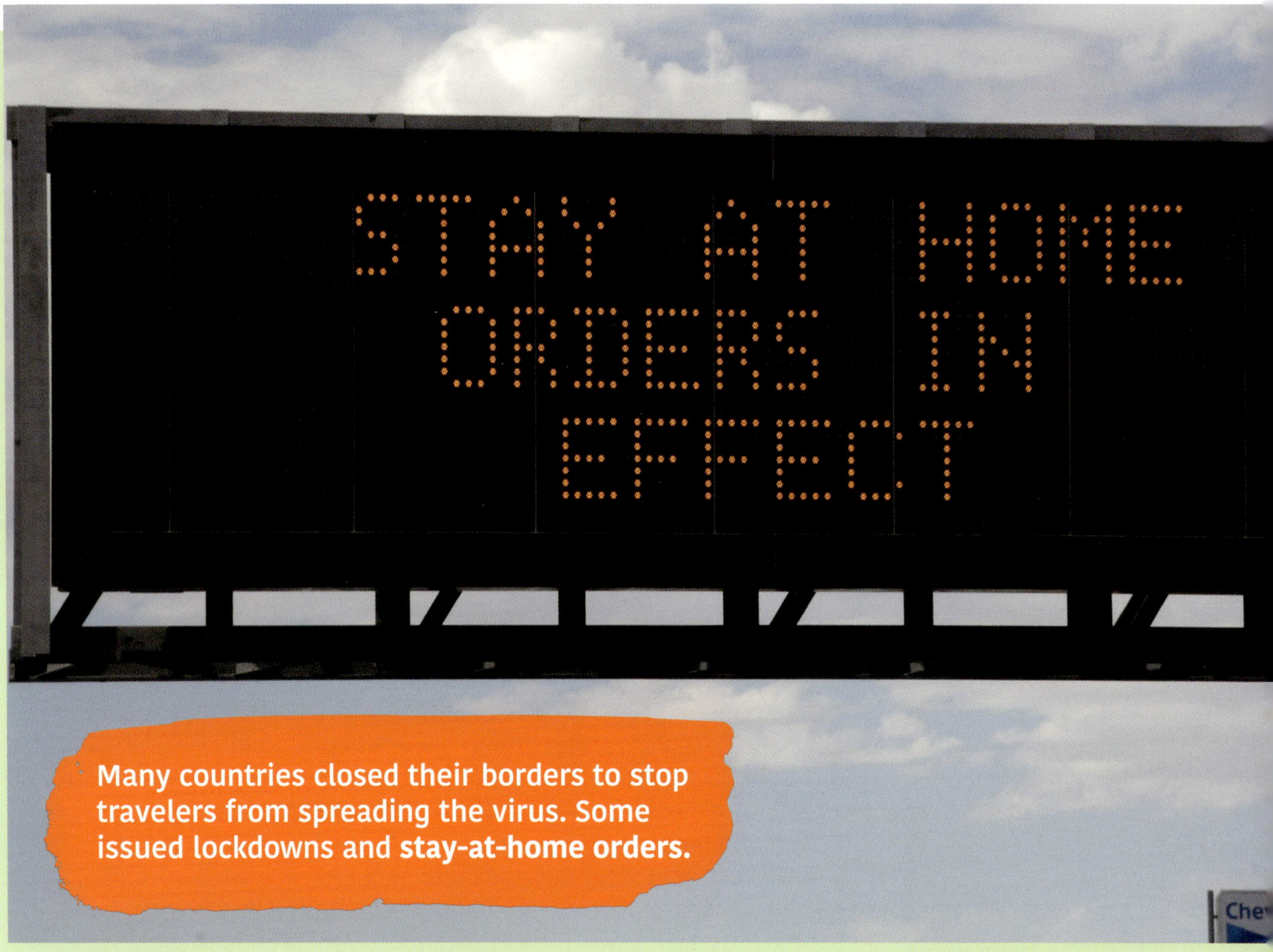

Many countries closed their borders to stop travelers from spreading the virus. Some issued lockdowns and **stay-at-home orders.**

The United States

The **World Health Organization (WHO)** labeled COVID-19 a pandemic on March 11, 2020. At that time, it had spread to 110 countries. In those first weeks, the U.S. government monitored the disease through its public health agencies and the **Centers for Disease Control (CDC)**. The virus was already circulating when the first case was confirmed in the United States on January 12.

National Emergency

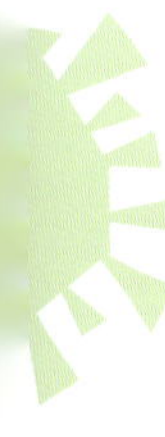

President Donald Trump declared a national emergency on March 13. This provided federal funding, or money, to help fight the disease. Travel bans were issued, hospitals geared up for **influxes** of sick patients, and industries and scientists began working on treatments and vaccines. But there was no national lockdown. Instead, state, city, and county governments set rules for lockdowns. That meant people in some parts of the United States were living their lives as normal, while others were not allowed to leave their homes except for emergencies. That difference also occurred between counties and communities within the same state.

California issued a stay-at-home order on March 19, 2020. It banned gatherings and closed schools, restaurants, and **non-essential** stores and services. Face coverings were required in public. Several other states followed. Some locked down for a month, others for more.

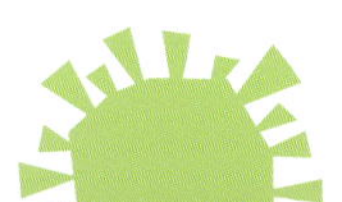

Canada

The first COVID-19 case in Canada was reported on January 25, 2020. By March 6, the country's **Minister** of Health suggested people start **stockpiling** food and medication. Twelve days later, Canada had 656 confirmed cases. Most provinces were on some sort of lockdown or stay-at-home order. The lockdowns forced many businesses to close, pushing people out of work. The Government of Canada set up financial supports for businesses and people. Lockdowns continued throughout the pandemic, with each province setting their own restrictions. Some had several lockdowns that were lifted when the numbers of infections were lowered.

The east coast provinces of Nova Scotia, New Brunswick, Prince Edward Island, and Newfoundland and Labrador created an "Atlantic Bubble." People who lived in those provinces could travel between them unrestricted. But anyone coming from other provinces had to **quarantine** for 14 days, just like they were coming from another country. That kept the number of infections in that area low for more than a year.

CITY OF PORT COQUITLAM
CORONAVIRUS (COVID-19)
HELP STOP THE SPREAD & STAY SAFE!
SPORT COURTS
CLOSED
until further notice
The City's priority is protecting the health and safety of residents and staff and to continue to serve you.

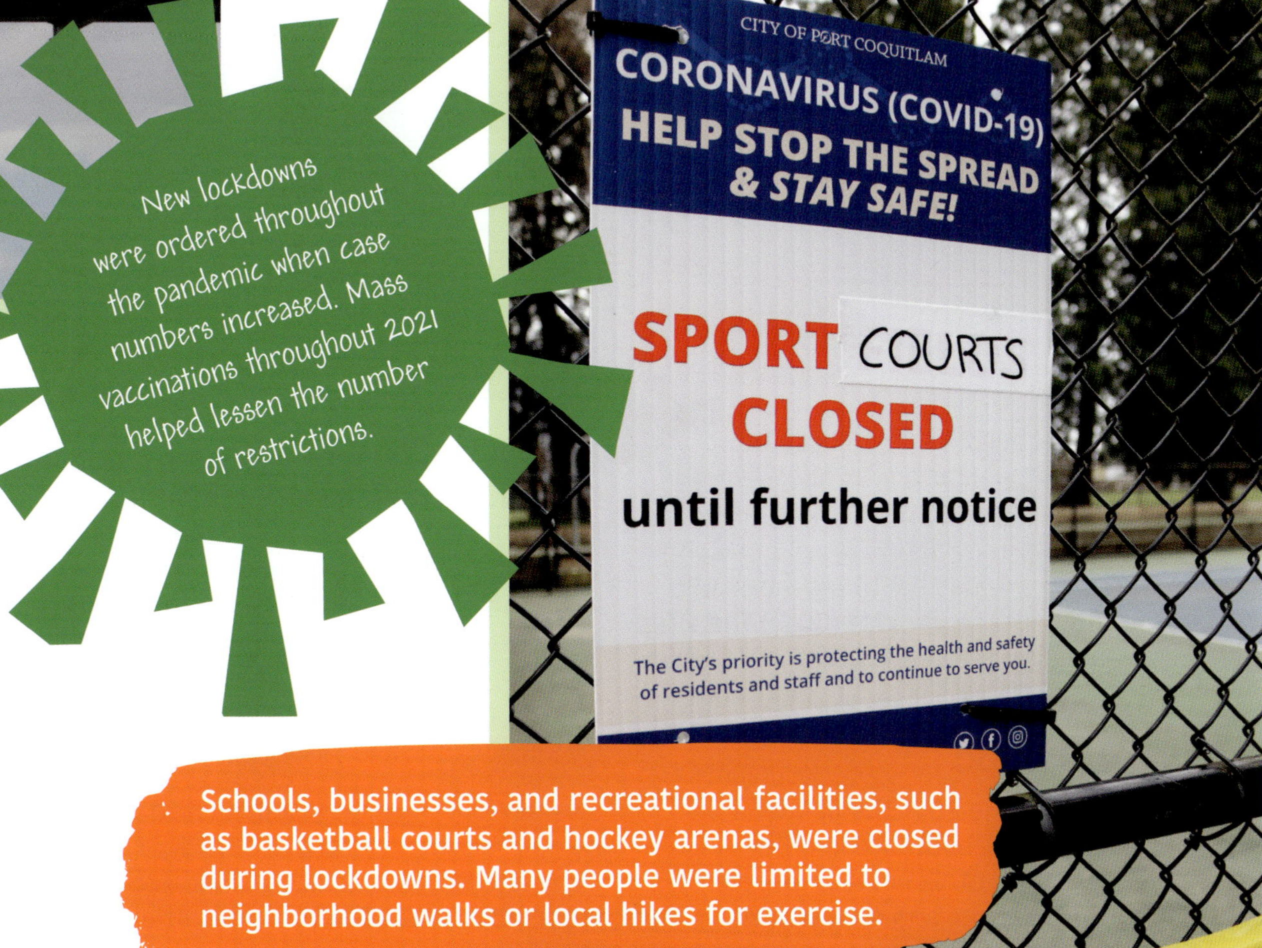

New lockdowns were ordered throughout the pandemic when case numbers increased. Mass vaccinations throughout 2021 helped lessen the number of restrictions.

Schools, businesses, and recreational facilities, such as basketball courts and hockey arenas, were closed during lockdowns. Many people were limited to neighborhood walks or local hikes for exercise.

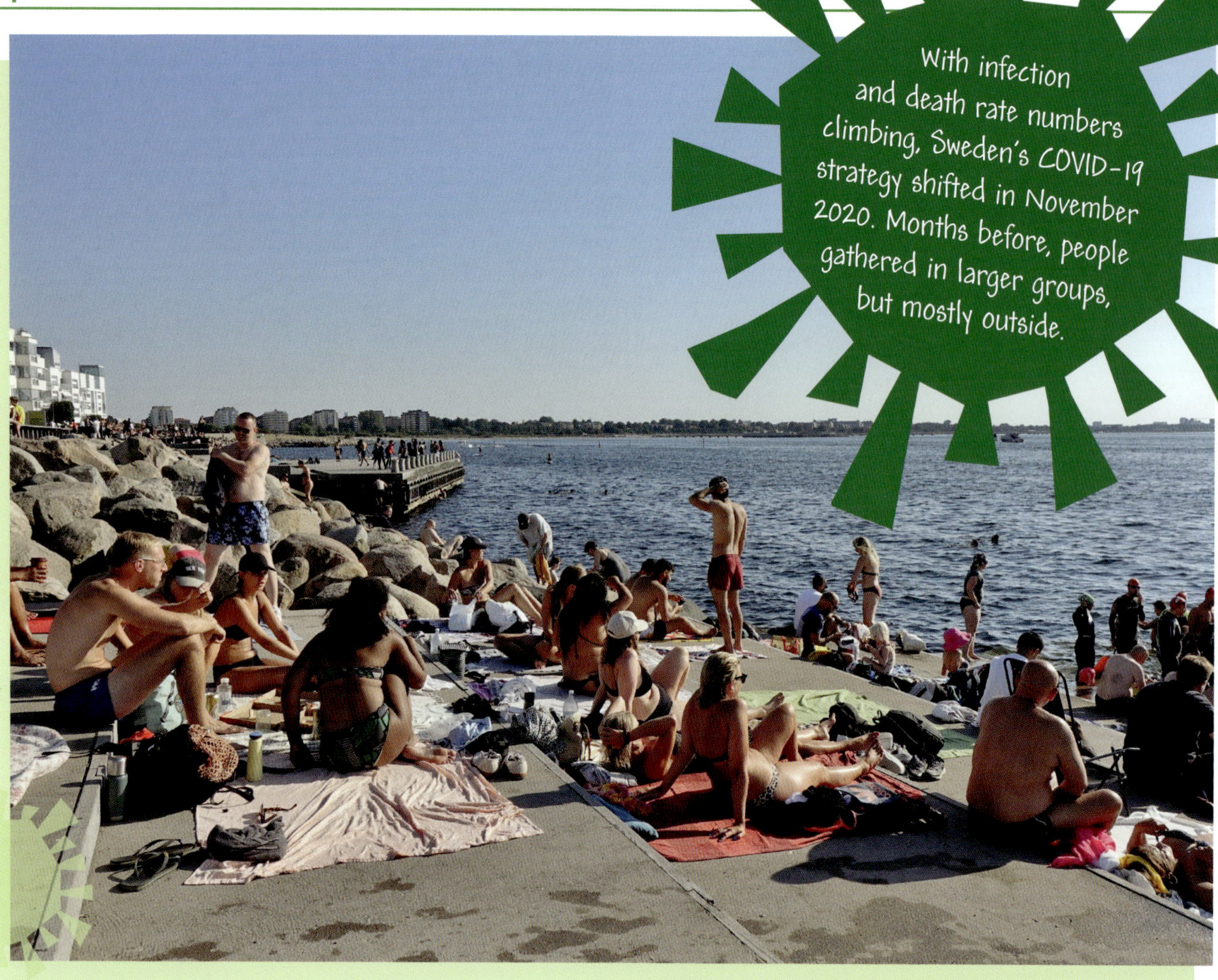

With infection and death rate numbers climbing, Sweden's COVID-19 strategy shifted in November 2020. Months before, people gathered in larger groups, but mostly outside.

No Lockdown?

There were some countries that chose not to lock down their populations at all. Their strategies for slowing the spread of COVID-19 did not include closing businesses and keeping people at home. That seemed to work for some countries at first. But as the pandemic wore on, many of those countries began to rethink their strategies.

Sweden's Method

In the early days of the COVID-19 pandemic, everyone was talking about Sweden. The Scandinavian country of 10.3 million people kept schools, gyms, bars, and restaurants open. Instead of a lockdown, the government attempted to flatten the curve a different way. The laws of the country meant the government could not legally impose a lockdown on entire regions or cities. It instead chose to ban large gatherings and events. It also asked people to adapt how they lived to halt the spread of the virus. Swedes largely followed a voluntary lockdown. They increased their hand washing, practiced social distancing, and worked from home if possible. But there were no laws put in place to make sure that happened.

Sweden had a higher COVID-19 death rate than its neighboring countries of Norway, Finland, and Denmark. But its businesses and economy did better than most European countries that were in lockdown.

Belarus

With most of Europe under lockdown and COVID-19 cases soaring in neighboring Russia, the eastern European country of Belarus was operating with a "business as usual" approach. The president of Belarus denied the severity of COVID-19. He told his people that it was nothing to worry about. Businesses were open, celebrations were encouraged, and the country's national football, or soccer, league continued to attract large crowds.

Few Regulations

Without direction from the government, the people of Belarus eventually began to practice social distancing voluntarily. For example, though Belarus was the last country in Europe to continue hosting live soccer games, the attendance dropped significantly as people in the country began to isolate themselves. In December 2020, Belarus began offering the Russian-made Sputnik V vaccine to its citizens. At that time, the country of 9.5 million people reported 1,400 deaths and 190,000 cases. By spring 2021, Belarus had put some restrictions in place. They included limiting attendance at events, such as soccer matches at 50 percent of stadium capacity. Restaurant tables also had to be set 6 feet (2 m) apart.

Volunteers made masks and face shields to give to health care workers in Belarus. Downplaying of the virus meant that health care workers faced a shortage of Personal Protective Equipment (PPE).

Over 4,000 people attended a Belarus Premier League soccer match on May 20, 2020. Most of them did not wear masks. In other areas of the world, professional soccer matches were canceled during the early months of the pandemic.

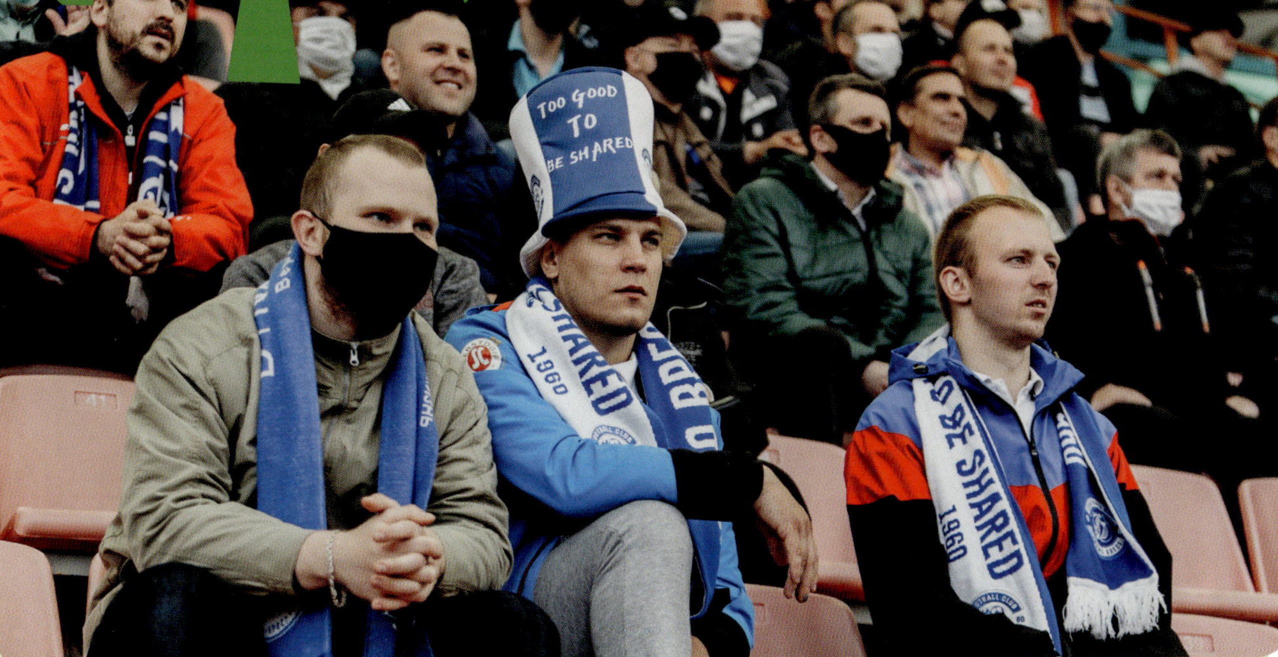

Lockdown Lifestyles

The COVID-19 lockdowns turned millions of people's lives upside down. The changes happened very quickly. In some areas of North America, many families and kids were getting ready for school and making plans for spring break—only to have schools canceled and travel restricted the next day.

Schools Closed

Most lockdowns around the world included some form of school closure. In many places, teachers and students had very little warning that changes were to come. Many went home for a regular weekend, then didn't return to school for months. When future generations look back at that period in time, school shutdowns are likely to stand out.

From March to May 2020, an estimated 55.1 million American students in public and private schools were sent home to build a new routine for learning. In Canada, most schools were closed by the end of March, 2020. Many schools reopened in September for the next school year, only to have to close again when infection rates went up.

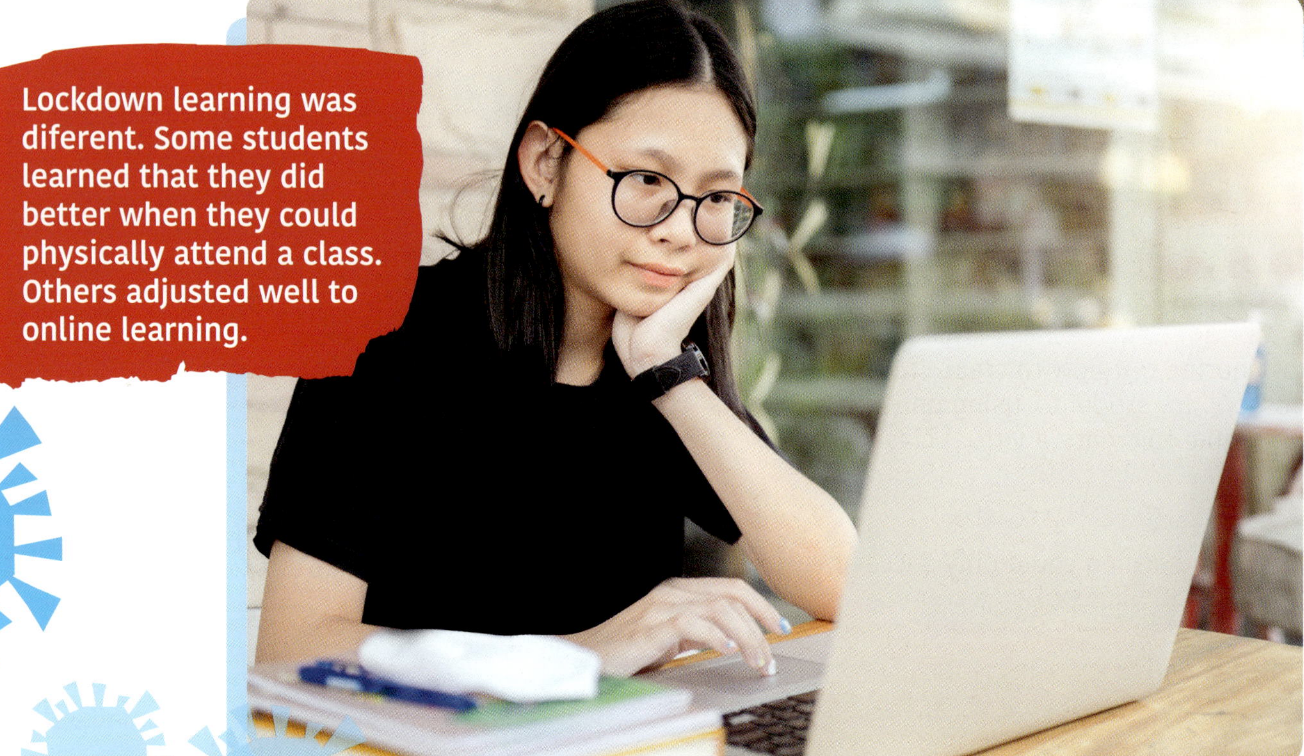

Lockdown learning was diferent. Some students learned that they did better when they could physically attend a class. Others adjusted well to online learning.

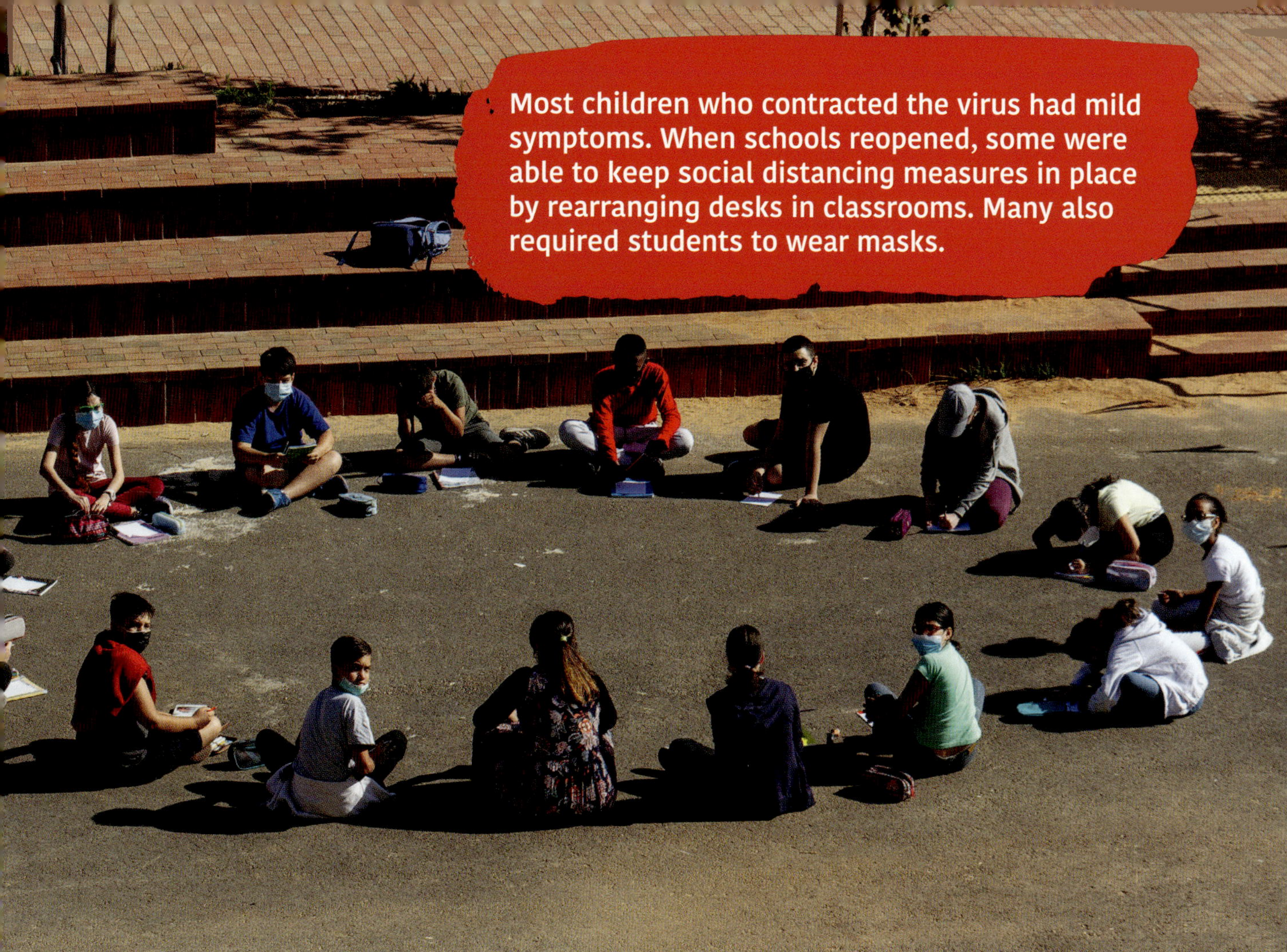

Most children who contracted the virus had mild symptoms. When schools reopened, some were able to keep social distancing measures in place by rearranging desks in classrooms. Many also required students to wear masks.

Remote Learning

Learning from home was challenging. It wasn't easy on young people who had to adjust to attending class on a computer. It wasn't easy on parents and caregivers who had to balance teaching from home and working to support their families. Teachers also had the difficult task of figuring out how to create fun and educational lessons for students, using one of many tools available to create a virtual classroom.

Learning Inequality

Remote learning could only succeed if students had access to computers, tablets, and reliable Internet. These things were much harder for some families than for others. For example. roughly 1.5 million people in New York City could not afford Internet at home. In Toronto, Canada, 38 percent of households reported Internet speeds below national targets in 2020. That became a major issue for online learning. The uneven access is called digital inequality. A U.S. government poll showed that nationwide, children in lower income households used paper lessons sent home from school. Some stopped school-based learning entirely.

Return to School

When schools reopened, most used a system recommended by health experts. Called the cohort model, the system had fewer students attending school in small groups called cohorts. The cohorts attended school in staggered schedules. Attending school in cohorts limited the number of contacts a student had. They did not mix groups of students or share materials. That lowered the chances of virus transmission.

Remote Work

When lockdowns started, students were not the only people who had to learn to do their work from home. Many workers realized that their jobs could be done quite well at home. Meetings could be held through live video and work could be shared through email. However, many people could not do their jobs from home. They were called **essential workers**. The closure of many businesses meant that a lot of people lost their jobs as well. Some governments provided financial help to citizens who lost their jobs due to the pandemic.

Essential workers were people employed by industries and businesses that did not close down. This included doctors, nurses, and other healthcare workers. It also included bus drivers, grocery store workers, delivery drivers, factory workers and more.

New Ways to Work

When public health agencies asked people to work at home if possible, the day-to-day lives of millions of people changed. Millions of people were used to waking up early to get ready for work, then hopping in their cars or catching public transit to travel to work. Instead, their morning commute was only a few feet away. Many people now worked from a kitchen table, basement, or bedroom–wherever a makeshift workspace could be made.

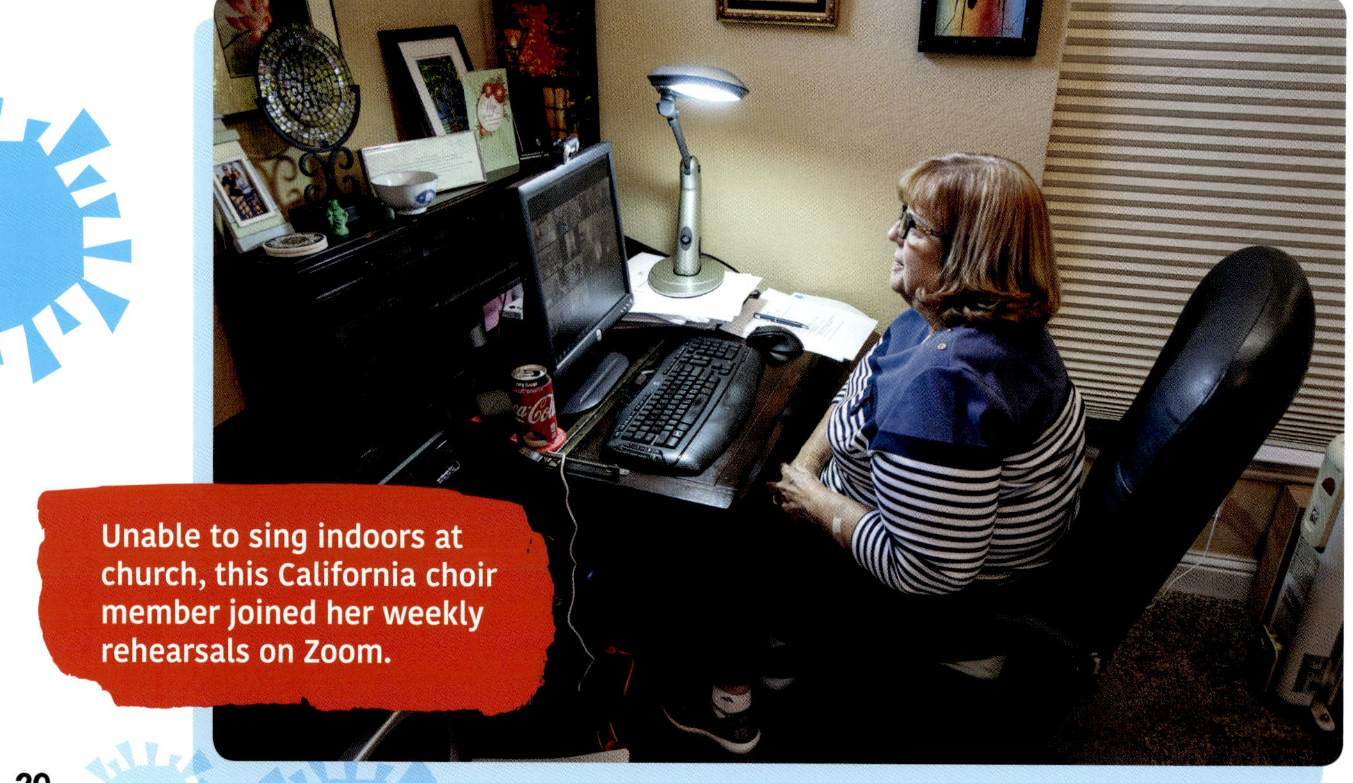

Unable to sing indoors at church, this California choir member joined her weekly rehearsals on Zoom.

PANDEMIC WHO'S WHO

Public Health Officers

Before the pandemic, hardly anyone knew who their local, state, provincial, or national public health officers were. During the pandemic, these leaders in public health became household names. Alex M. Azar II was the United States Secretary of Health and Human Services when COVID-19 emerged. He declared it a public health emergency for the entire country on January 21, 2020. He pushed for quick treatments and vaccines to tackle the virus. Azar was replaced by Xavier Becerra in March 2021. Becerra expanded the vaccine program. He worked alongside Dr. Anthony Fauci, who was chief medical officer to several presidents. Dr. Fauci was a well-known face on television. He answered media questions on COVID-19 and reassured the public. Canada's national health officer, Dr. Teresa Tam, also appeared on television regularly to answer questions. She advised the federal government on pandemic strategies. Each province had its own chief public health officer. All of them were medical doctors, and most of them were women. British Columbia's chief provincial health officer, Dr. Bonnie Henry, was admired for her calm and kind announcements of new illness numbers and deaths. Dr. Henry even had a shoe named after her! The bright-pink Mary-Jane shoes made by John Fluevog Shoes have Dr. Henry's "be kind, be calm, be safe" motto stamped into them.

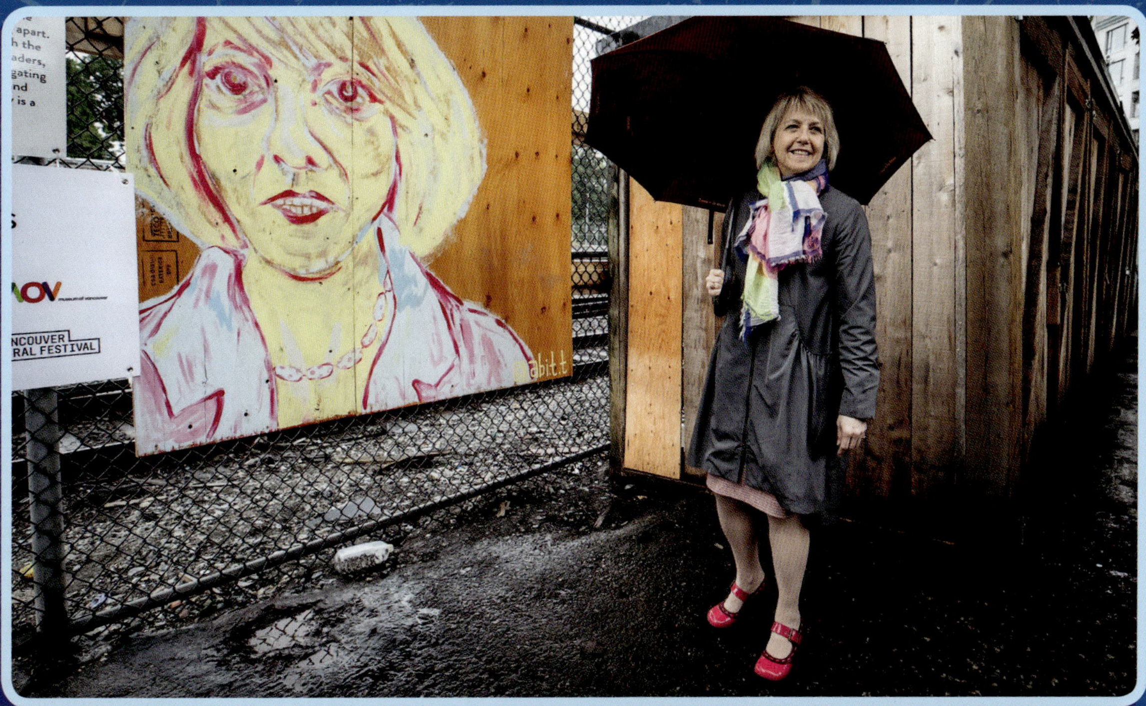

Dr. Henry's pink shoes sold out right away. They were later produced in other colors. The company donated 100 percent of its profits from the shoe to the charity Food Banks B.C. Then, 15 percent of later sales went to the WHO COVID-19 Response Fund.

The Demand for Delivery

During lockdowns, grocery stores remained open and people were allowed to leave their homes to buy food. However, many were afraid to shop for groceries in person. That created a new demand for services such as grocery delivery and curbside pickup. In the early days of COVID-19, grocery delivery services were backed up for weeks. Many families were preplanning their grocery purchases carefully to make sure that each food delivery or trip to the grocery store went a long way.

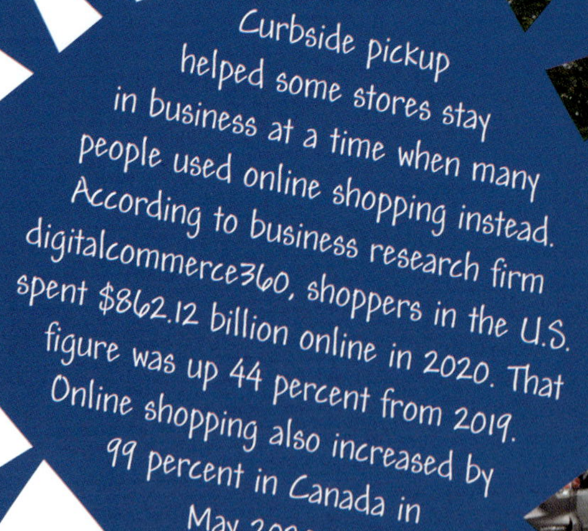

Curbside pickup helped some stores stay in business at a time when many people used online shopping instead. According to business research firm digitalcommerce360, shoppers in the U.S. spent $862.12 billion online in 2020. That figure was up 44 percent from 2019. Online shopping also increased by 99 percent in Canada in May 2020.

Restaurants Change Tactics

Most lockdowns banned in-person dining at restaurants. Restaurants were allowed to stay open for takeout and food delivery, though. For many families, ordering takeout from a restaurant was at the top of a very short list of things that could make life feel more "normal." Takeout was a way to keep restaurants in business while still keeping people safe. The concept of takeout was soon applied to retail stores, as curbside pickup became another pandemic trend. Even with takeout to help, the National Restaurant Association in the United States said the food service industry lost $240 billion U.S. in sales in 2020. Almost 2.5 million jobs were also lost. Many restaurants closed for good. According to the Canadian restaurant association, Restaurants Canada, an estimated $44.8 billion was lost over the first year of the pandemic.

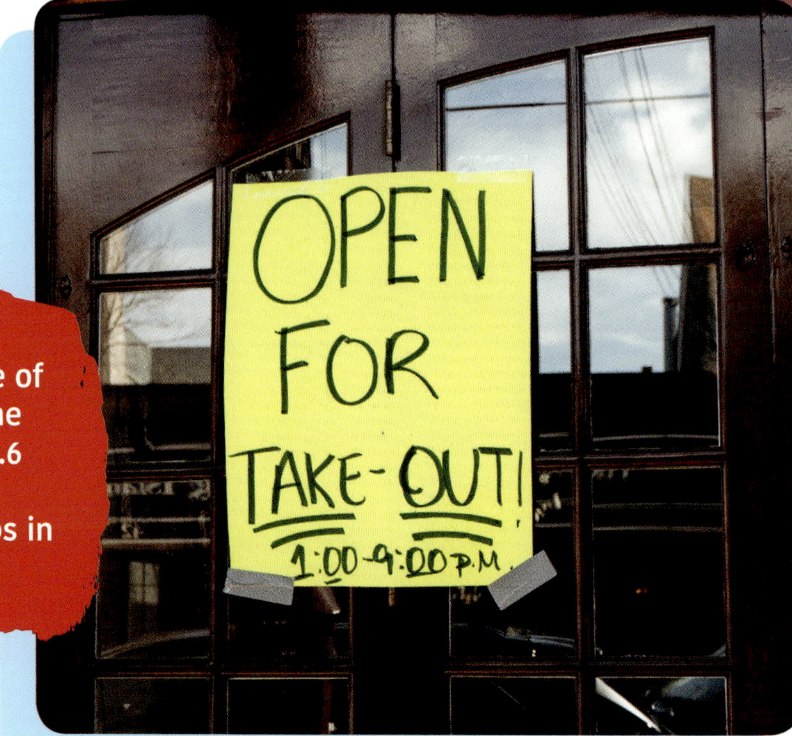

The restaurant and food service industry was one of the hardest hit during the pandemic. It provides 15.6 million jobs, or about 10 percent of all payroll jobs in the U.S. economy.

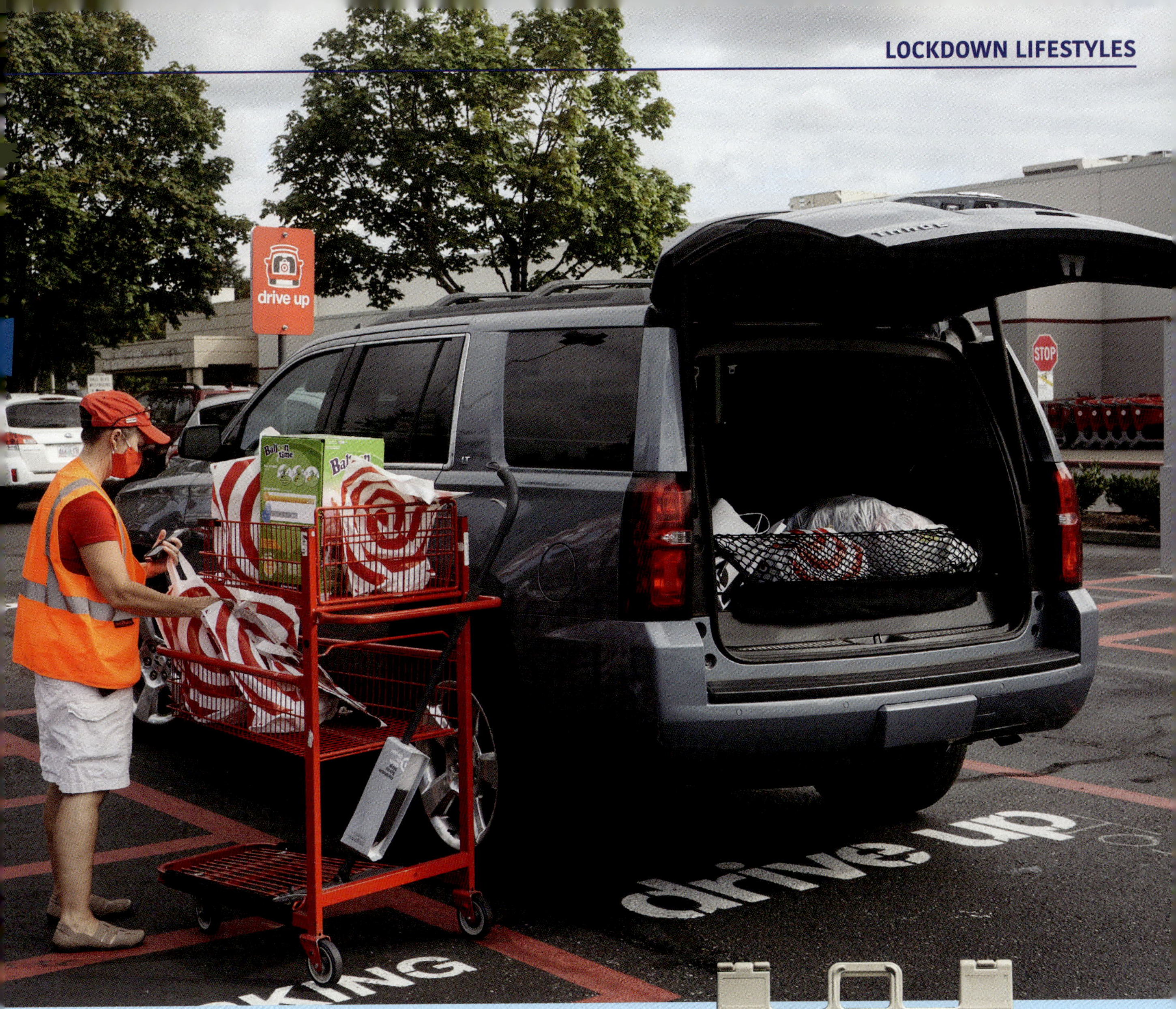

Retail Changes

Once the initial strict lockdowns began to lift, retail stores began to open. Still, for many, it was only for curbside pickup. Curbside pickup meant ordering a product online or over the phone, and arranging for a specific time to pick up that product outside the store. Stores set up specific curbside pickup parking spots for customers. Often, customers were told to text a special number when they arrived. Then, a store employee would run the item out to the customer's car. Curbside pickup allowed stores to stay open and people to shop safely. One of the biggest difficulties for retail stores and restaurants was repeated lockdowns and reopenings. With each lockdown, they had to adjust their **business models** and staff numbers.

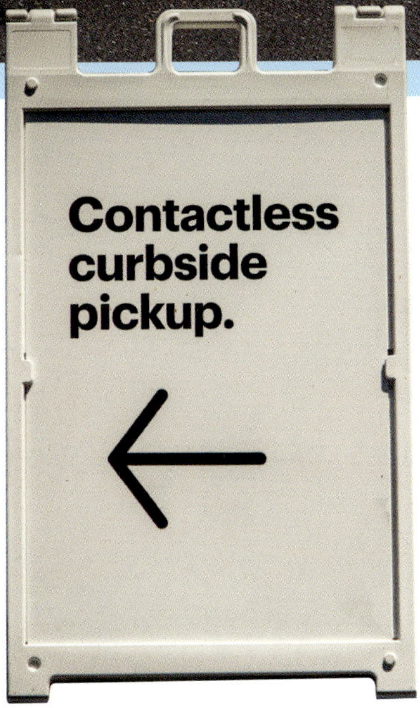

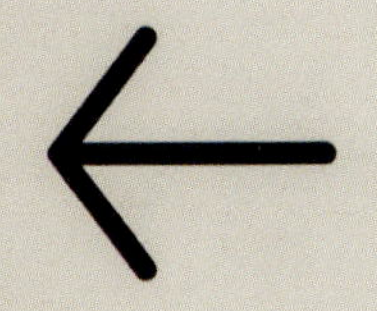

Chapter 3

Pandemic Problems

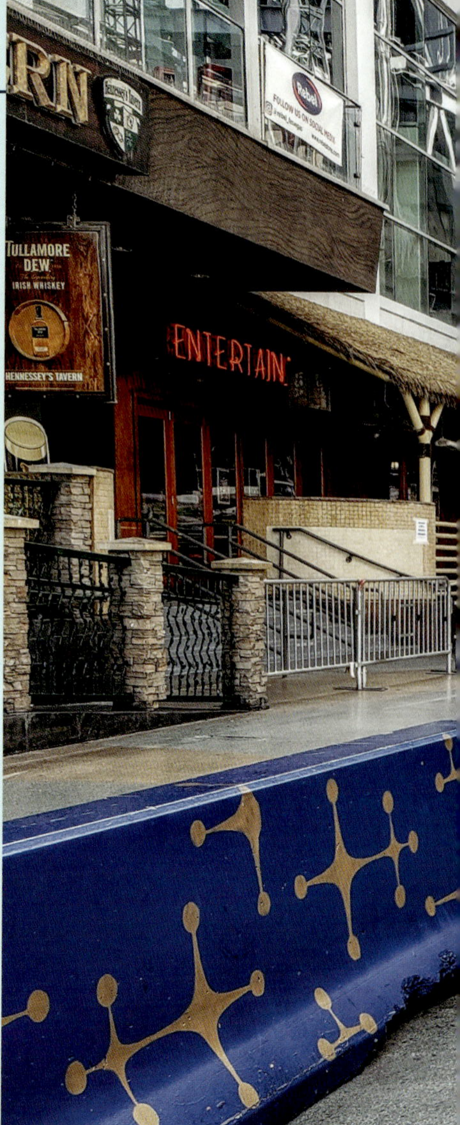

As businesses closed during the lockdowns, millions of people lost their jobs. There was a sudden shutdown of **consumer** activity. Some areas had stay-at-home orders that allowed people to leave their homes only for necessary work, food shopping, or emergencies.

Pandemic Unemployment

The spring of 2020 was a very challenging time for the workers of the world. In February 2020, 6.2 million Americans were unemployed. In just three months, that number more than tripled to 20.5 million people. These were the people who lost jobs because of the pandemic. The biggest rise in unemployment was felt by workers younger than 25 years old. The pandemic affected young people more because they often work in industries that were hit hardest by the lockdowns, such as retail and hospitality, which includes restaurants, hotels, and entertainment. Before the pandemic, 12.6 percent of 16-to-19-year olds were unemployed in the United States. By May 2020, 29.9 percent of workers in that age group were unemployed. Many went back to work when the worst of the pandemic was over.

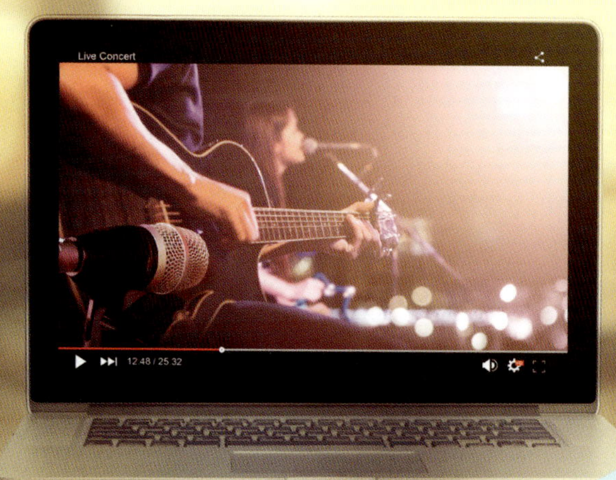

Musicians and entertainers lost large parts of their incomes during the pandemic. Live concerts, shows, and plays were shut down. Many shifted to offering online concerts to fans for small fees or donations.

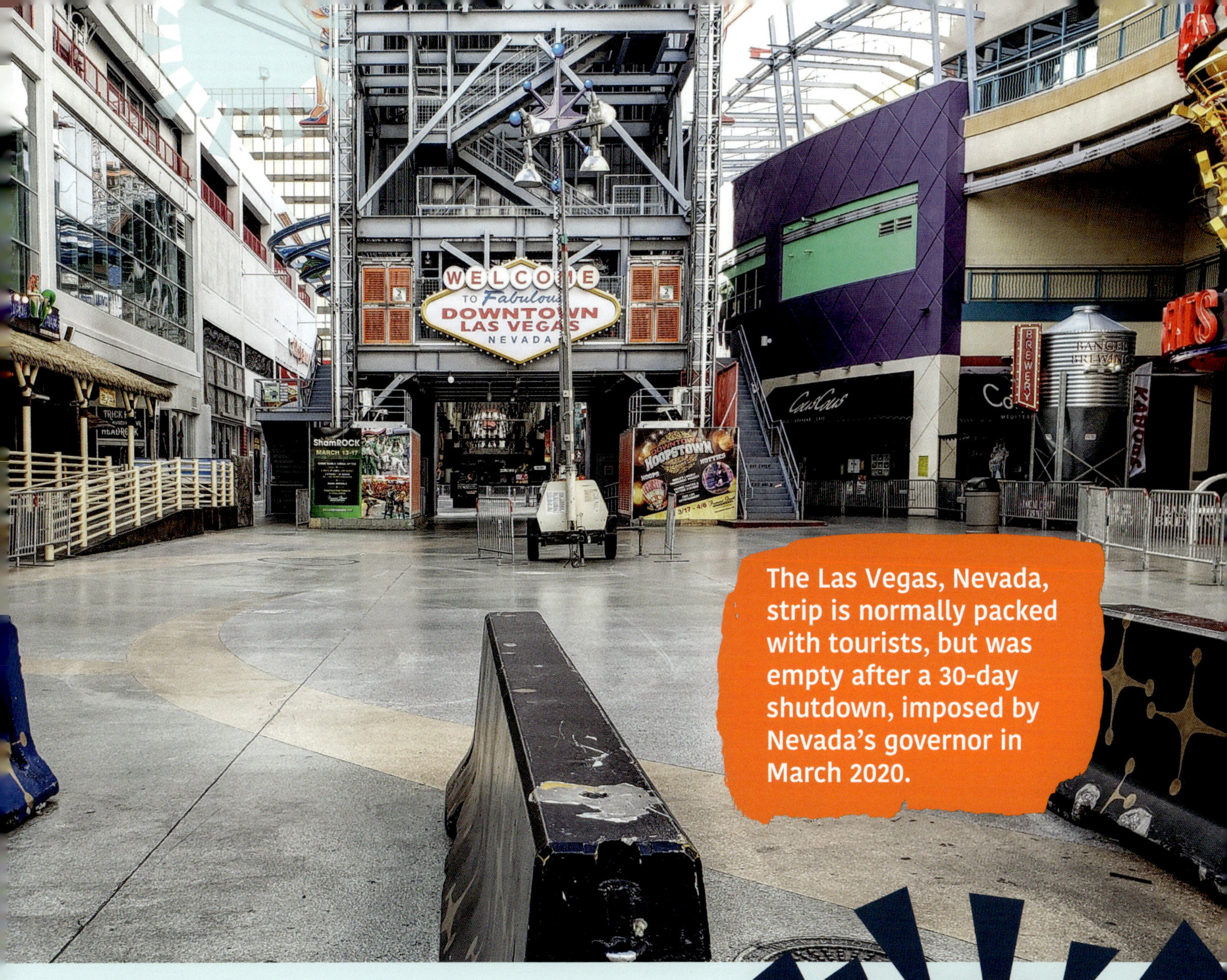

The Las Vegas, Nevada, strip is normally packed with tourists, but was empty after a 30-day shutdown, imposed by Nevada's governor in March 2020.

Less Money, Less Spending

Even people who hadn't lost their jobs changed their spending habits during the pandemic. The uncertainty of the pandemic made people fear the future. Those who had the ability to save, saved more. In February 2020, Americans were saving about 8 percent of their income. By March, that number had jumped to 33 percent. It was a positive thing that people had money to save and were thinking about their financial future. But it also meant less money was being spent at local stores, restaurants, hotels, and other businesses. Those were hard hit by the COVID-19 pandemic. Some hotels and motels stayed open by becoming shelters. Cities and service organizations rented the rooms to handle overflows of **unhoused** people at regular shelters. Some businesses were unable to find new ways of making money. Many closed permanently.

In some cities, small motels and hotels were repurposed. Some were used as shelters for unhoused people. Others became quarantine centers for people returning after living or vacationing abroad.

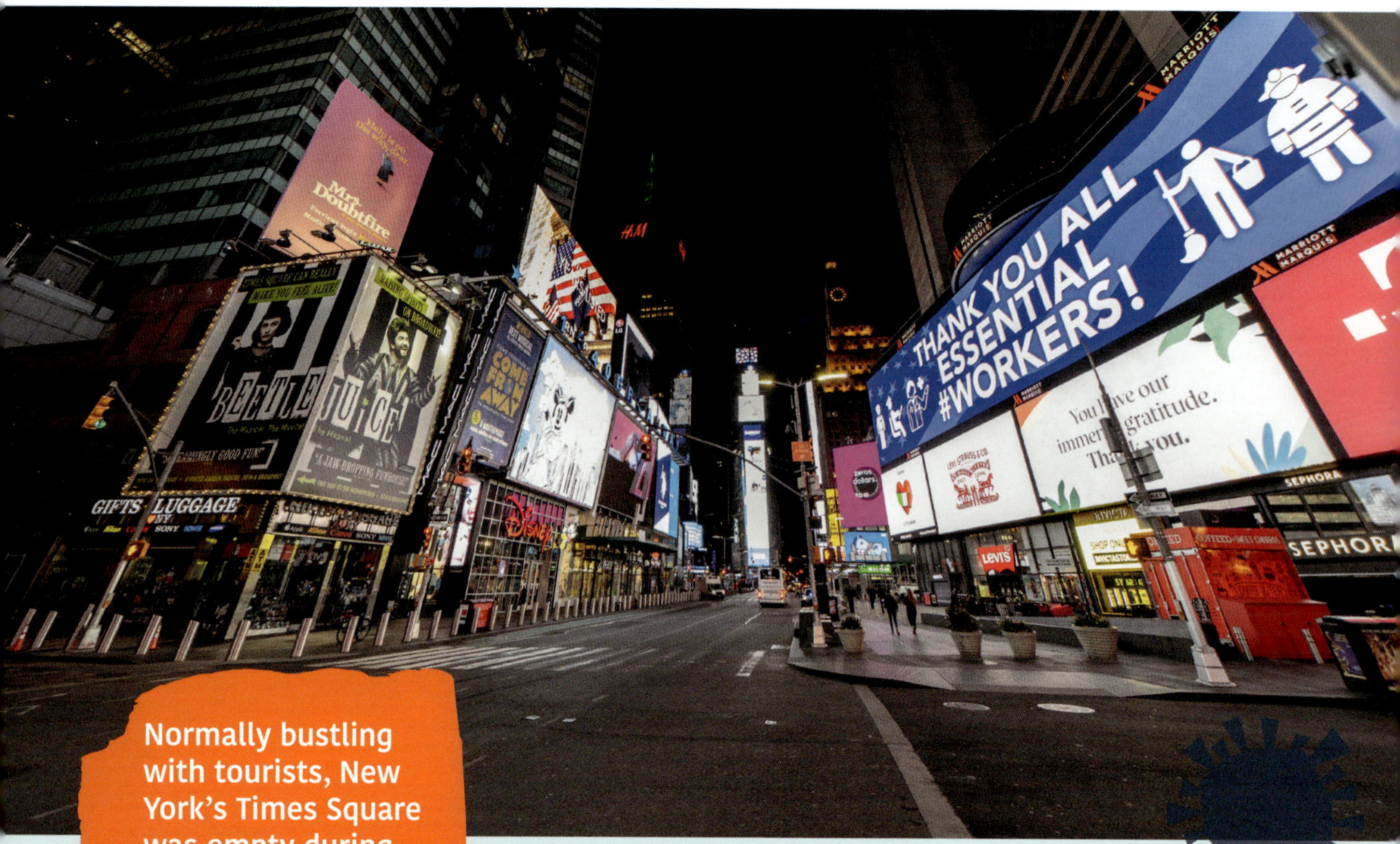

Normally bustling with tourists, New York's Times Square was empty during the first pandemic lockdown in April 2020. The city's famous Broadway theaters were closed for 18 months. That pushed actors and all theater workers out of work.

Hard-Hit Industries

The industries hardest hit by COVID-19 lockdowns were hospitality and retail. International borders closed around the world and people were often restricted from traveling within their own countries. That devastated the travel industry. In 2019, the tourism industry accounted for 10.2 percent of the world's **gross domestic product (GDP)**. That means millions of people work in that industry and were at risk of losing their livelihoods.

Hotels Take a Hit

The hotel industry was feeling the pain caused by the lockdowns. Even in cities where hotels were allowed to stay open, bookings were low. People often had no reason to travel. Many didn't feel safe staying in hotels during a pandemic, either. The sudden, drastic cut in the number of people who were traveling caused massive unemployment. Millions of people employed by hotels, airlines, buses, trains, and cruise lines around the world were out of work almost instantly. The World Travel & Tourism Council, a travel industry research organization, estimated that the travel industry lost up to 197 million jobs and reduced global GDP by up to $5.5 billion. The final tolls won't be known for years.

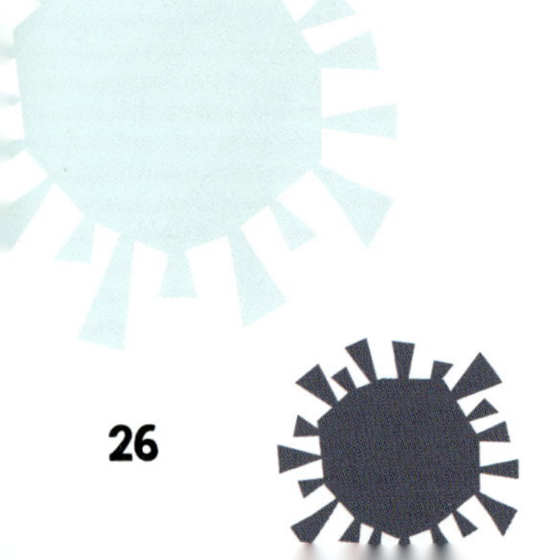

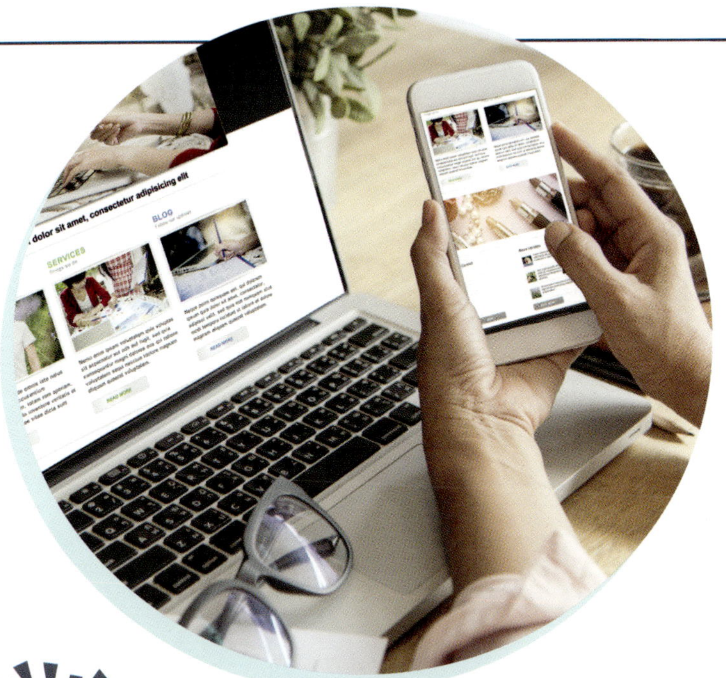

Shopping Changes

The retail industry was hit hard by COVID-19. In-person shopping was viewed as risky and unnecessary, and most lockdowns included restrictions on retail stores. In many areas, retail stores were completely closed. Larger retailers relied on their online shopping sites. Smaller stores—those owned by people who live and work in a community—were forced to change the way they did business. Many spent money developing online sales. Some also focused on promoting their businesses on social media, with online videos and forums with buyers.

PANDEMIC WHO'S WHO

Jacinda Ardern

The COVID-19 pandemic proved that leadership matters when a country is faced with a new and life-threatening disease. On March 14, 2020, the island nation of New Zealand had six known cases of COVID-19. But its leader, Prime Minister Jacinda Ardern, decided to "go hard and go early" with the pandemic response. Ardern put border restrictions in place early. She made it mandatory for people coming home to New Zealand to self-isolate. Her government also put money into pandemic response and stressed community **collaboration**. That included testing high-risk groups and setting up a National Health Coordination Centre. New Zealand had seen the desperation of medical workers in Italy and Spain during the pandemic's **first wave**. Ardern was determined her country would not go through that. On March 23, 2020, Ardern put the country of 5 million people into a three-month lockdown. Schools were closed. Guided by teachers, students were allowed to work from home at their own pace. The country opened up when COVID-19 numbers went down. Life almost returned to normal. By spring 2021, New Zealand had one of the lowest COVID-19 death tolls at 26. That made it one of the safest countries during the pandemic.

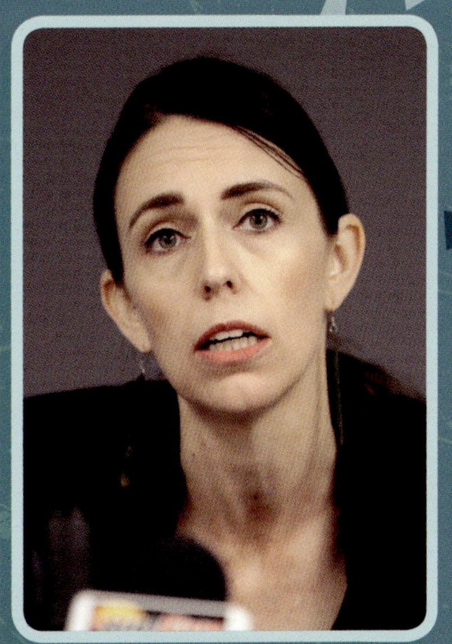

Jacinda Ardern and her party were re-elected to government in October 2020 elections. Voters felt she was a good leader during the middle of the pandemic.

Lockdown Mental Health

The COVID-19 pandemic gave people a sense of uncertainty that most had never experienced before. No one knew how, when, or if it would end. At the beginning, the main source of fear and **anxiety** in North America was the virus itself. It was a new disease tearing across China and Europe. People could see that many were infected and hospitals were finding it hard to cope with the numbers of sick and dying patients. Government lockdowns were difficult for people to live through. Often when the lockdowns were eased or ended, the virus came back. People lived for happy moments but often, the news brought more things to worry about. Months passed with the virus surging in waves. Some countries had two and three waves before a vaccine was produced to protect people from the virus, and **mass vaccinations** started. Some countries had few vaccines and had to wait for other countries to donate them.

Loss of Routines

Beyond the virus, another major cause of worry was the effect lockdowns had on children. School closures impacted the mental health of children, youths, and their parents in a major way. For kids and youths, closing schools meant a big change in routine. That was devastating for those with mental health challenges or special education needs who relied on the structure and services offered at schools.

Parents and caregivers were trying to balance working from home with playing the role of teacher to school-aged children. That created stress, anxiety, and exhaustion for everyone.

Lockdowns and school and work closures meant that kids didn't spend their days with friends anymore. They didn't hang out, have dinner with their grandparents, or go to parties. This left many people feeling isolated and alone.

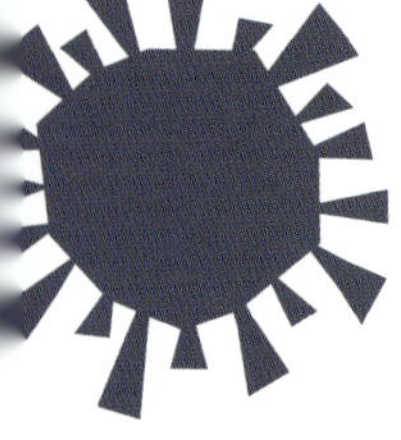

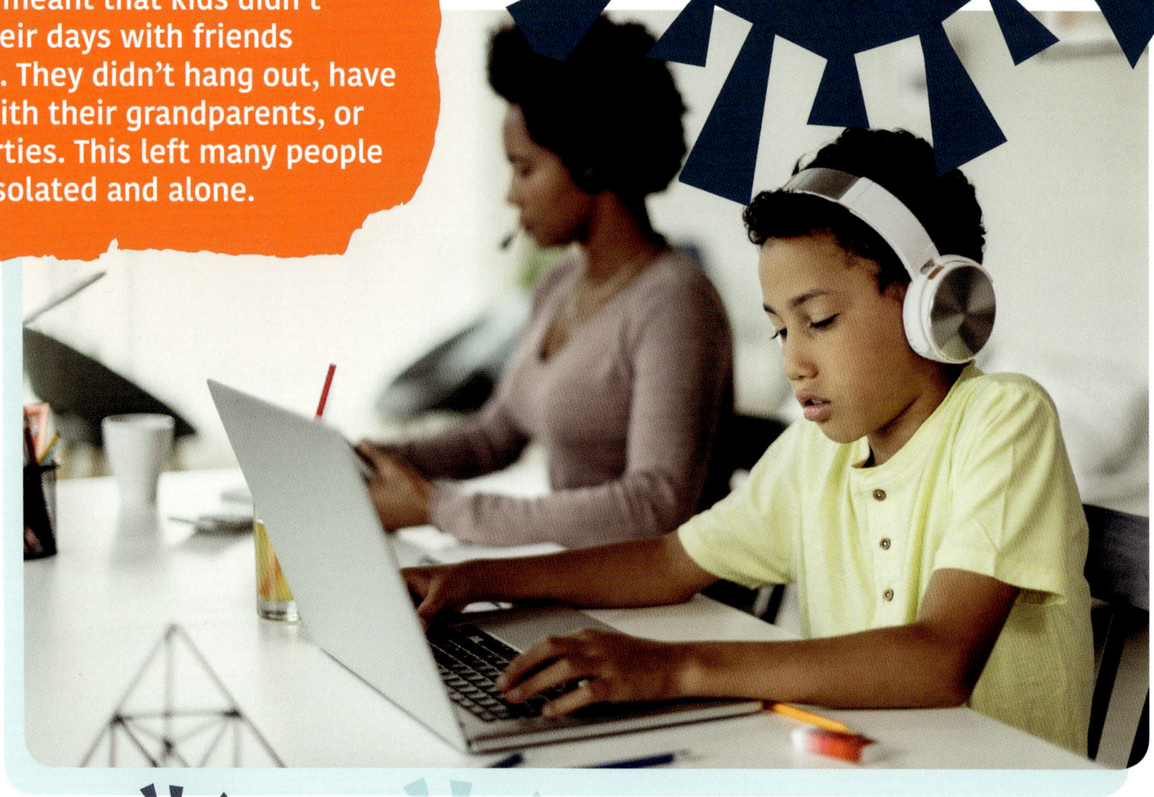

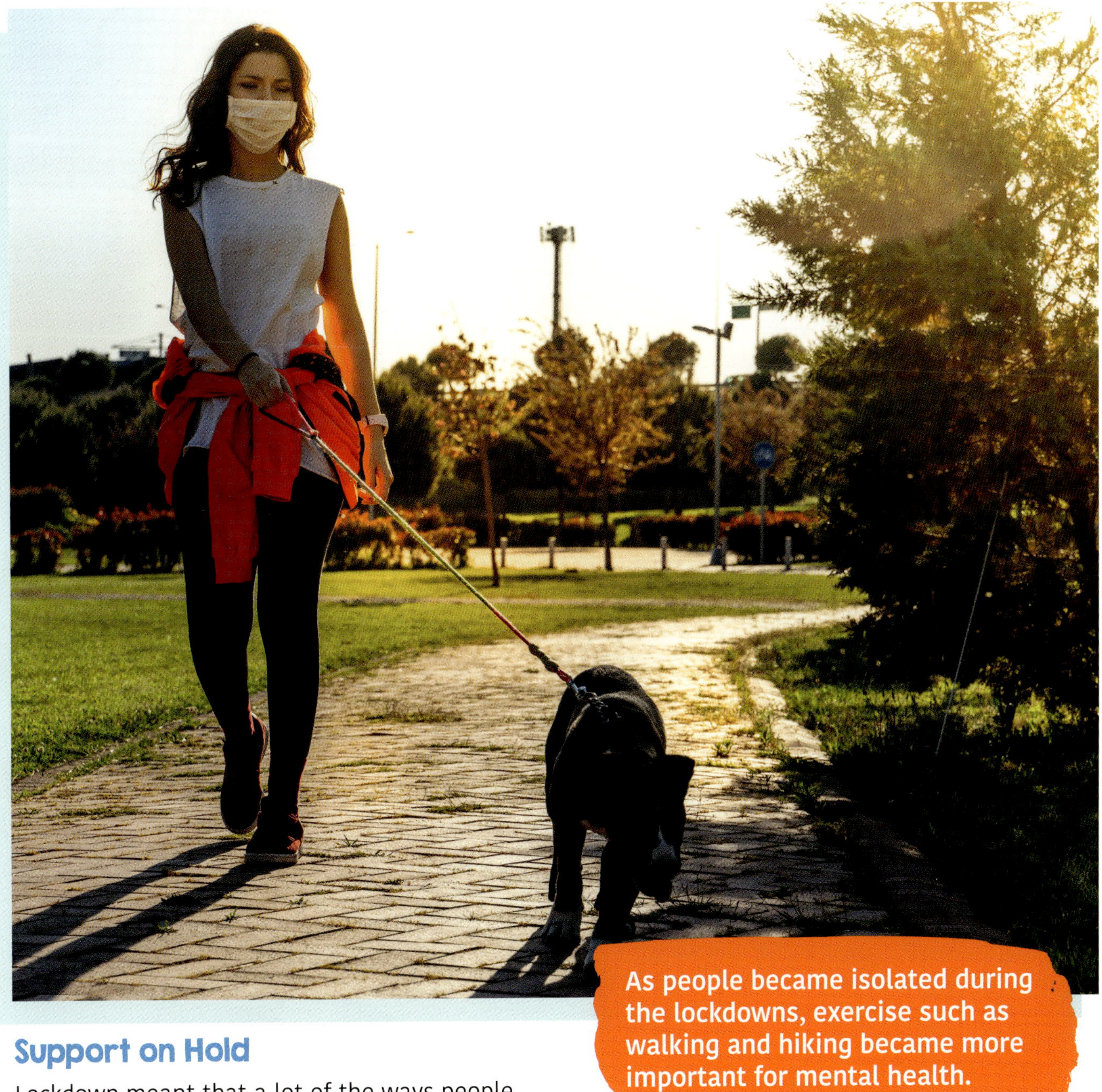

As people became isolated during the lockdowns, exercise such as walking and hiking became more important for mental health.

Support on Hold

Lockdown meant that a lot of the ways people coped with stress were unavailable or more difficult to access. Adults and children with mental health challenges before the pandemic faced new challenges without the supports they previously had. In the United Kingdom (U.K.), mass lockdowns meant about 26 percent of adults with mental health conditions were unable to access regular services. Support groups and "face-to-face" counseling stopped during lockdowns. Some people were able to get help online.

Anxiety and Depression

Depression and anxiety increased around the world during the pandemic. People mourned their pre-pandemic lives. In the United States alone, more than one in three adults reported symptoms of anxiety or depression during the pandemic. Essential workers, especially health care workers, were affected more negatively.

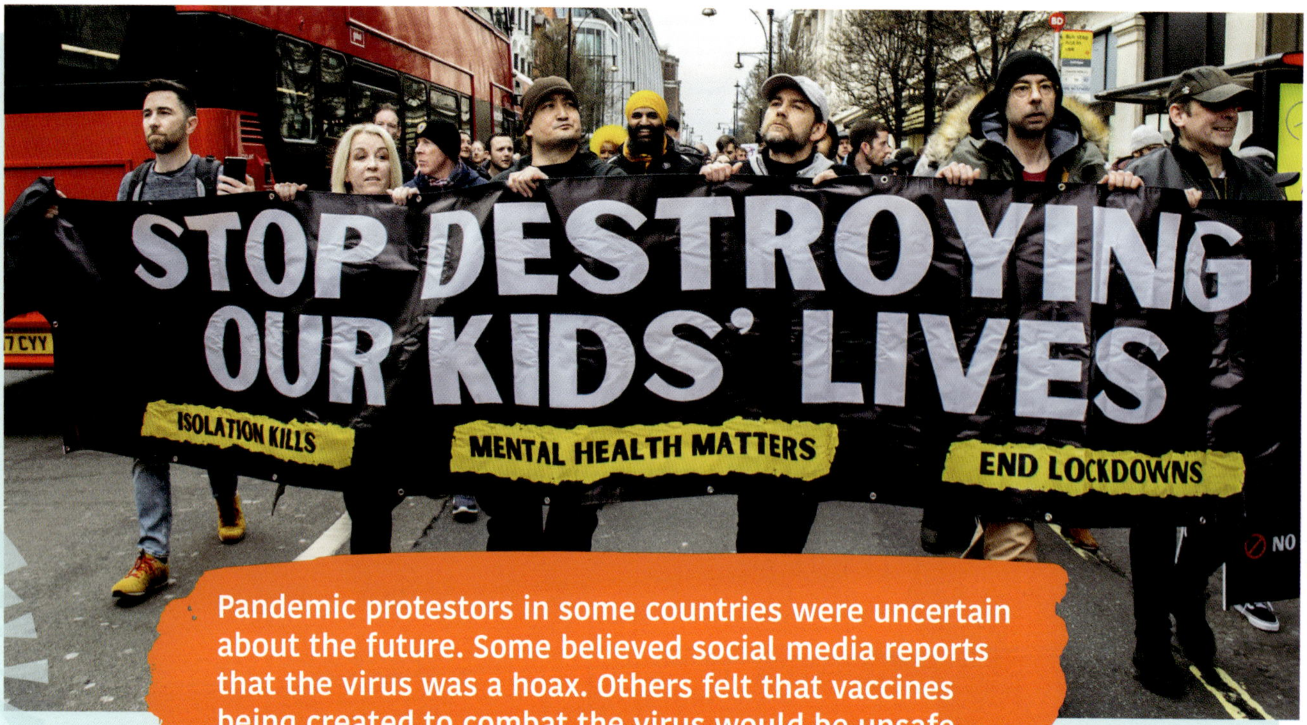

Pandemic protestors in some countries were uncertain about the future. Some believed social media reports that the virus was a hoax. Others felt that vaccines being created to combat the virus would be unsafe.

Lockdown Protests

Not everyone was willing to follow rules and regulations during the pandemic. Some people rejected the idea that COVID-19 was a serious disease that required everyone to work together to stop the spread of the virus that caused it. Others objected to the idea of governments reducing personal freedoms through lockdowns and other rules. In many parts of the world, people took to the streets to protest COVID-19 regulations. The protests became more common over time and as the number of lockdowns increased.

Out in the Streets

Many protests were driven by anger. Anti-mask protestors rejected the idea that masks could help prevent transmission of the virus. They refused to wear masks in public places such as stores. Anti-mask and anti-lockdown protestors feared the government was taking away their freedoms. Some formed groups that protested regularly in public spaces, such as parks and in front of government buildings. During non-lockdown periods, they protested in shopping malls. Their aim was to get the government's attention and draw people to their cause. In some countries, protestors were angry about losing jobs and incomes. In many countries, governments set up **income support** programs to help people who were out of work because of the pandemic. The money often wasn't enough. In poorer countries, those out of work had to look after themselves.

Protests became extremely common during the COVID-19 pandemic. By April 2020, there was approximately one significant, anti-government protest every four days.

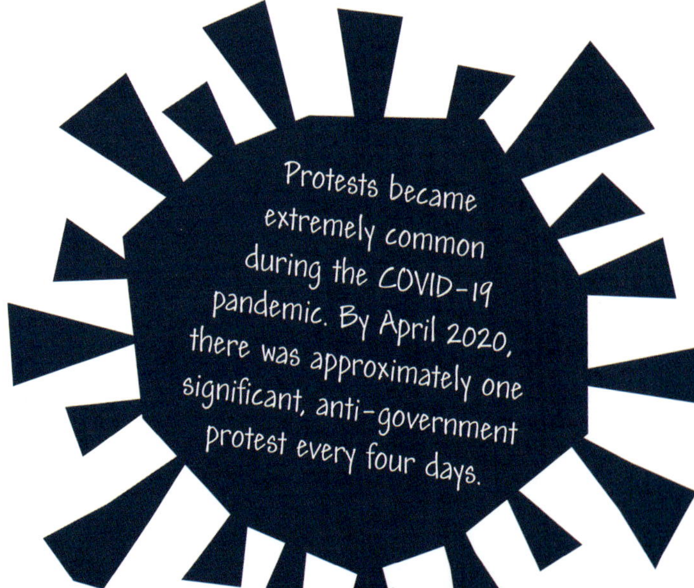

Not Doing Enough

Other protests involved people asking for more help and more resources to fight the virus. Early in the pandemic, health care workers struggled to find enough personal protective equipment (PPE), such as masks and gloves, to keep them safe while doing their jobs. Governments all over the world struggled to find and buy enough PPE. In some countries, such as Brazil, people protested because they felt their governments were not taking the virus seriously enough. These people were angry that their leaders were **prioritizing** the economy over the health of their people by keeping businesses open and avoiding lockdowns.

Mask Anger

Many people protested being told to wear masks. Some countries, such as the United States, Canada, and Russia had no national policy around the usage of face masks in public spaces. Many other countries, such as France, Colombia, Egypt, and South Africa, required people to wear a face mask while out in public.

Even in countries that had no national mandatory mask rules, individual cities, towns, states, and provinces had their own rules. And where there were rules around wearing masks, there were protests against them.

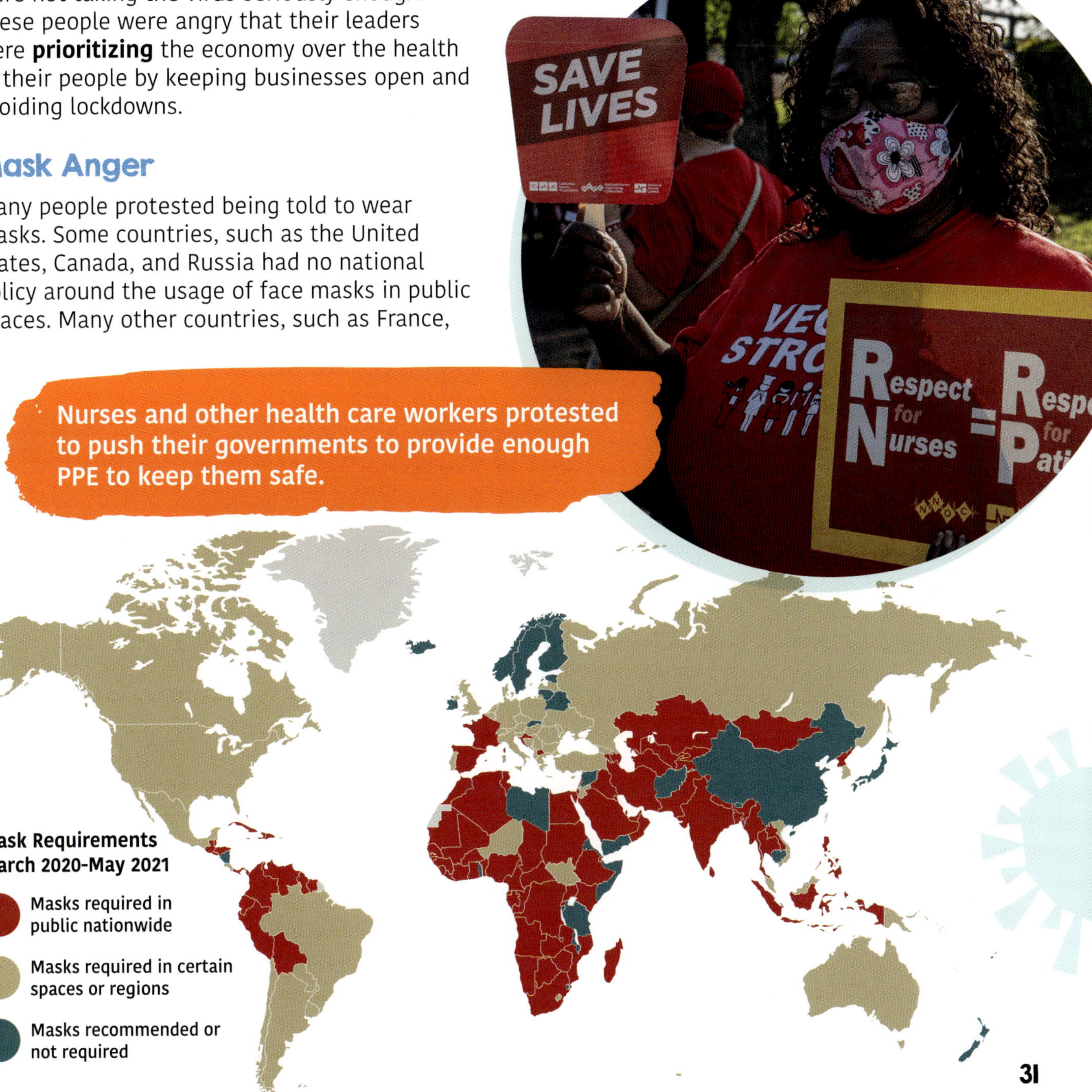

Nurses and other health care workers protested to push their governments to provide enough PPE to keep them safe.

Keeping It Social

Humans are very social. Most enjoy being around other people. Imagine not being able to hug your mom, open gifts with your friends on your birthday, or dance at your cousin's wedding. During COVID-19 lockdowns, many people couldn't do any of those things—for well over a year.

Getting Social Online

Rules about the number of people allowed to gather in one place seemed to change all the time. The numbers were usually different for indoor gatherings and outdoor gatherings. That is because scientists discovered it is harder to catch COVID-19 from a person outdoors. There, constant airflow helps to carry respiratory droplets away. In comparison, droplets tend to hang **stagnant** in the air indoors.

Sporting Events

COVID-19 canceled many mass gathering events, such as concerts and sports events. Many amateur sports were sidelined, but professional sports adapted. Many leagues shortened their 2020 seasons, grouped teams in "bubbles," and prevented fans from attending. The National Basketball Association (NBA) suspended its season in March 2020. It then restarted in July, when all 22 teams played their games in a bubble at Walt Disney World in Florida. Professional sports opened up more in the spring and summer of 2021.

Professional sports is big business. The NBA spent $190 million on building the 2020 season bubble for play. The investment paid off with an estimated $1.5 billion in income.

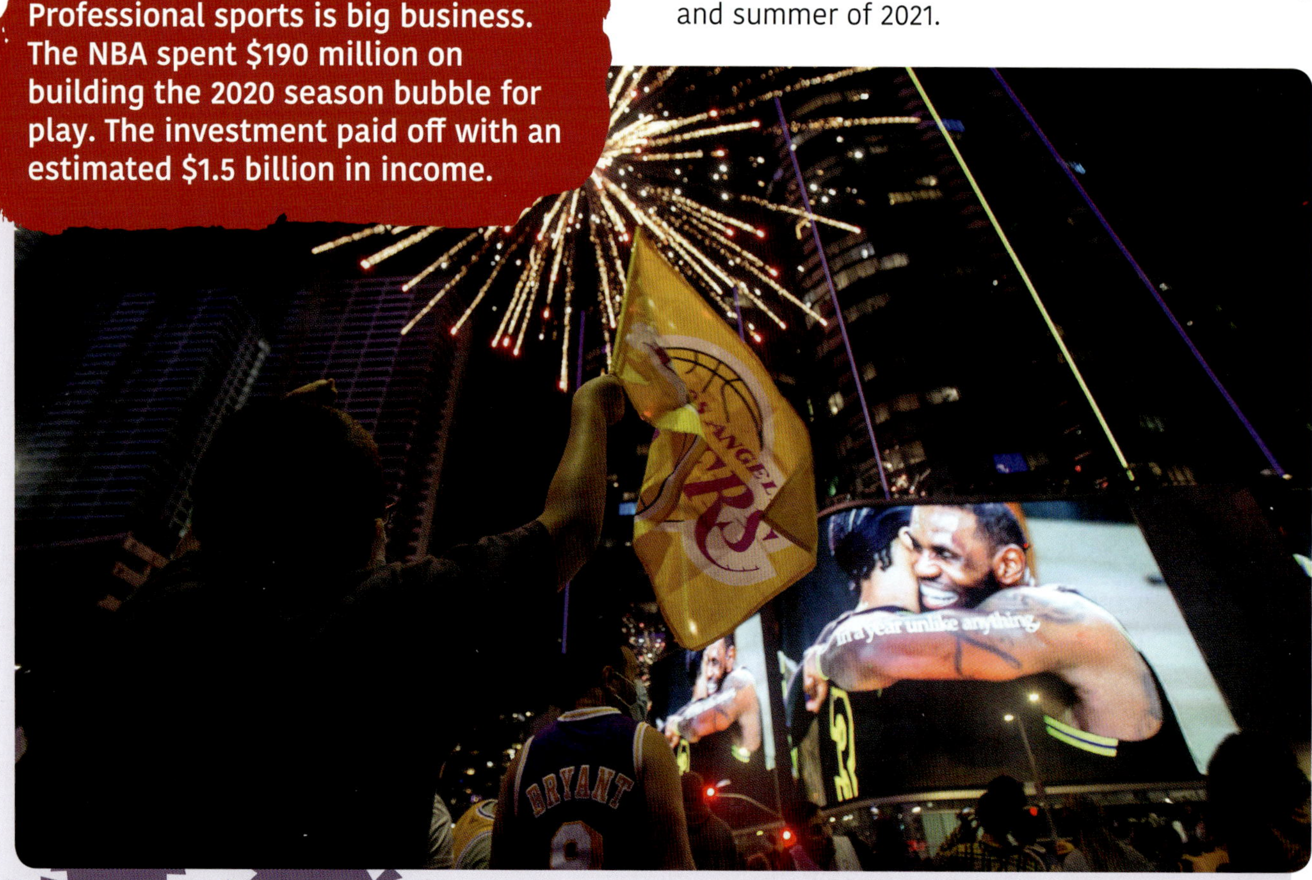

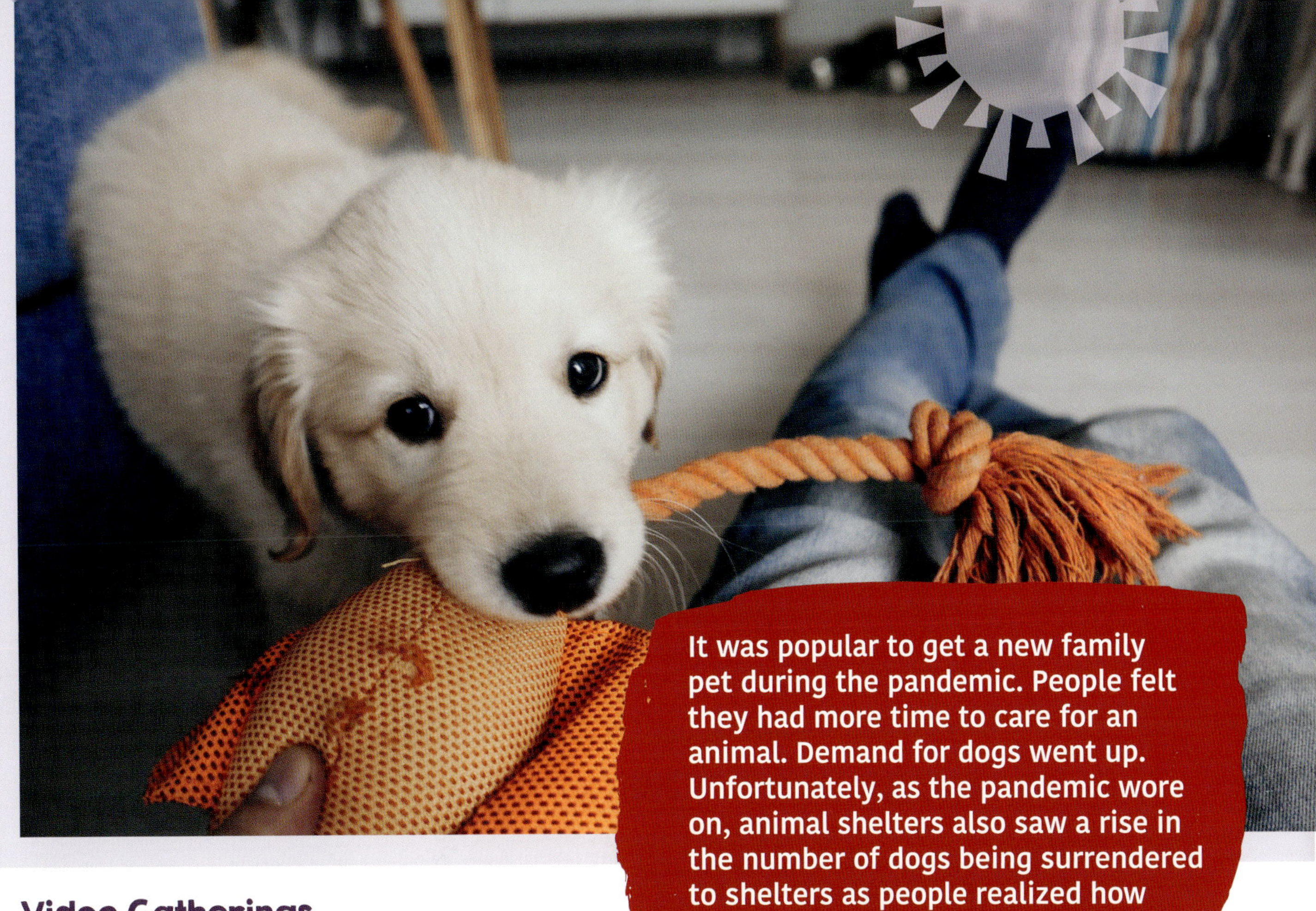

It was popular to get a new family pet during the pandemic. People felt they had more time to care for an animal. Demand for dogs went up. Unfortunately, as the pandemic wore on, animal shelters also saw a rise in the number of dogs being surrendered to shelters as people realized how much work pets could be.

Video Gatherings

Lockdowns were hard for everyone. Even professional athletes admitted that they felt odd and sometimes sad that they could not play in front of fans. Many people felt sad and lonely. Kids missed chatting with their classmates. Adults missed visiting with their friends and families. Grandparents missed playing with their grandchildren. Luckily, many people had access to computer technology. Video gatherings, in many cases, took the place of physical interaction.

Drive-By Events

Another way people stayed connected during the pandemic was with drive-by events. Drive-by birthday and graduation parties became a common occurrence in many neighborhoods. People stood outside their homes while their friends drove by, honking, cheering, and sometimes dropping gifts on the sidewalk. It was a creative way for people to celebrate life events with their friends, without the risk of spreading COVID-19.

For many people, online group chats became common Saturday night plans. Friends got together online to catch up, play a game, or have a simple conversation. It was an easy, safe way to be social, while also following the lockdown rules and staying healthy.

Pandemic Weddings

While it certainly seemed like it at times, the world did not stop when COVID-19 began to spread. People got engaged before the pandemic started, and they had weddings planned for 2020. Many postponed their weddings for another year in hopes that the world would be "back to normal" by then. Others decided to find a way to host a wedding safely, while obeying government restrictions.

Smaller Celebrations

When lockdowns were the strictest, people were not allowed to have any gatherings at all. Many people decided to get married outside, in backyards and parks. As lockdown restrictions changed, weddings changed, too. In some areas, restrictions meant weddings of fewer than 10 people attending were allowed. In other areas, weddings with fewer than 50 people were allowed. Small weddings had an effect on the wedding industry, or the businesses that support weddings. Photographers, caterers, wedding planners, and wedding venues lost jobs and income.

This couple planned a traditional wedding with 100 guests before the pandemic. New COVID-19 rules meant changing locations and cutting the guest list in half. So they switched to a small, backyard wedding.

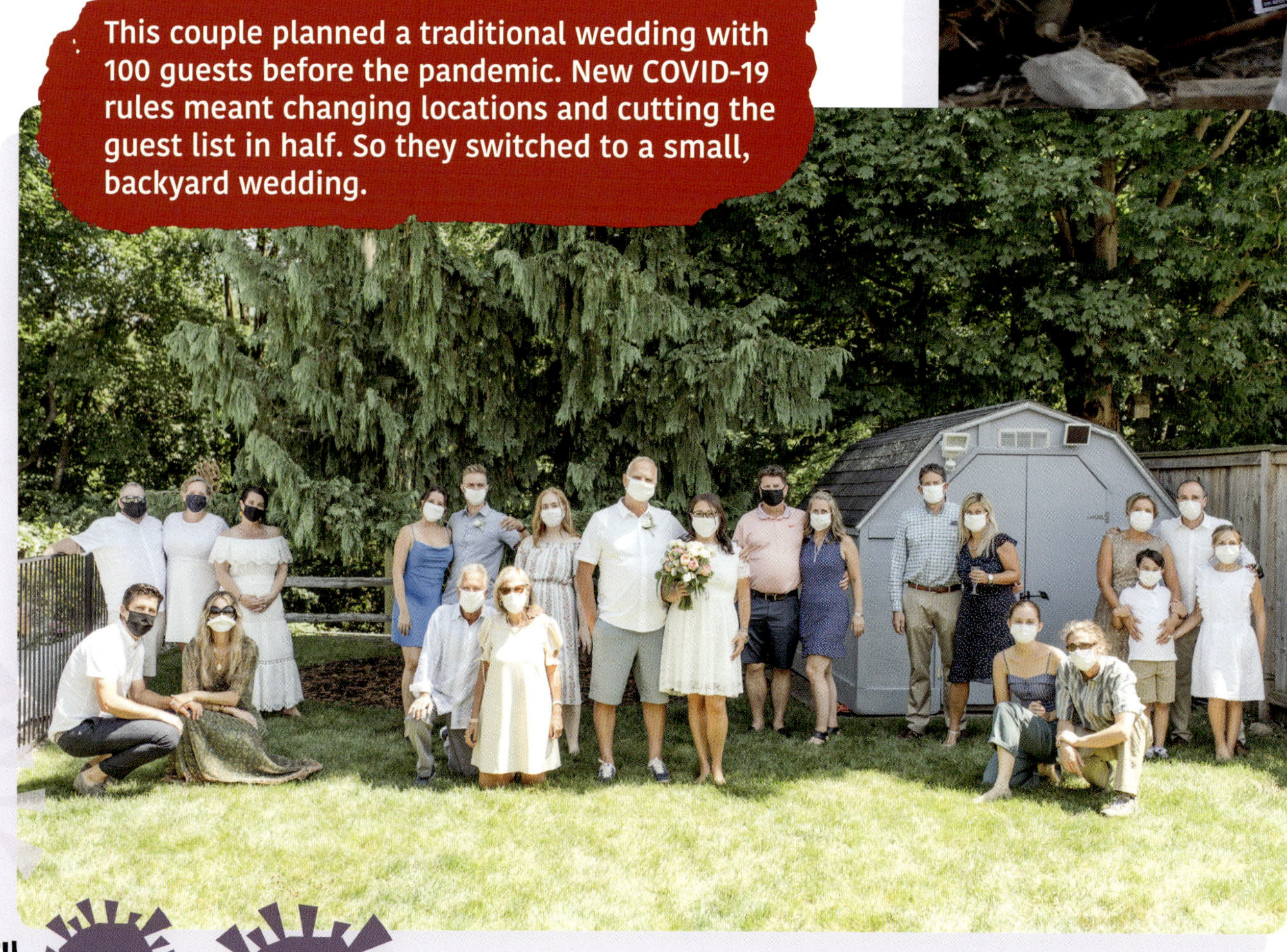

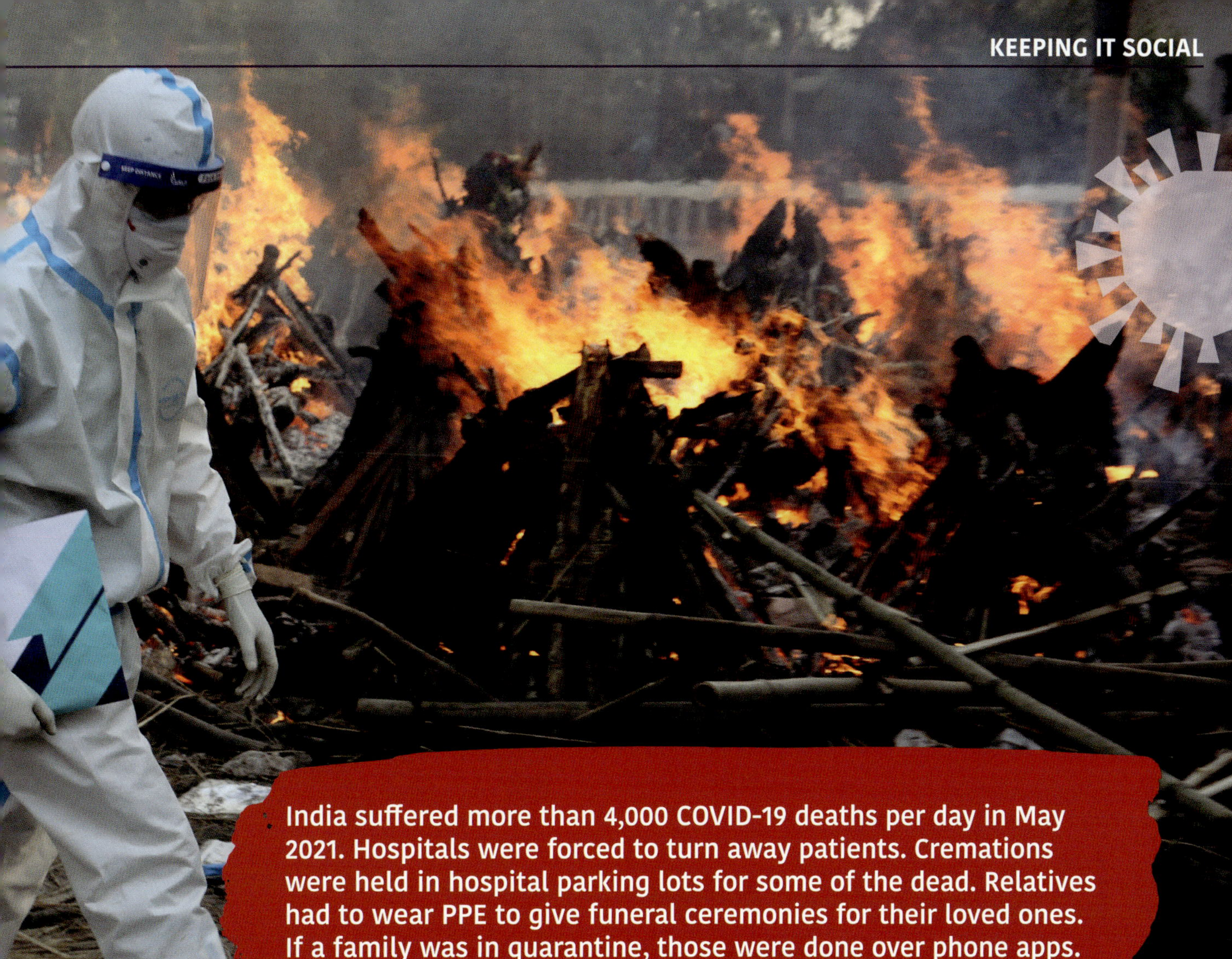

India suffered more than 4,000 COVID-19 deaths per day in May 2021. Hospitals were forced to turn away patients. Cremations were held in hospital parking lots for some of the dead. Relatives had to wear PPE to give funeral ceremonies for their loved ones. If a family was in quarantine, those were done over phone apps.

Funerals During COVID-19

While people continued to celebrate happy milestones such as weddings, sad occasions happened as well. Typically, people gather together for a funeral to share stories and pay respects to the person who has died. The pandemic changed the way people marked death. Funerals and other gatherings for mourning were an early source of virus transmission. Because they normally involve people praying, singing, hugging, or holding hands, they became dangerous contact events. Funeral homes and places of worship adapted funerals to be safer. Unfortunately, it meant small and often less-comforting final goodbyes. In some areas, pandemic restrictions meant only a few people could gather for a funeral. They had to be masked and socially distanced. In others, funeral homes set up walk-by or drive-by funerals where a limited number of people could pay their respects by viewing a closed casket. Some people chose to postpone funeral gatherings until a date when it would be safer.

Streamed Goodbyes

Like many other social events during COVID-19, some funerals took place online. Links to livestream the funeral service were sent out to friends and family before the event. Instead of attending in person, people logged in to share memories of the person who had passed away and to give each other support.

Lockdown Restrictions

While lockdown measures were put in place to keep people safe, they did make life more difficult. Many people were suddenly out of work because businesses were closed. People who were used to seeing their friends and family all the time were lonely. Some people, who did not believe that the virus was dangerous at all, felt the restrictions were unnecessary.

Breaking the Restrictions

For these reasons, many people decided not to follow the lockdown restrictions. They refused to wear masks. They continued to gather in groups. Some even had big parties. A few people opened their businesses, even though they were told they had to close. Every action has a consequence, and breaking lockdown rules was no different. Just like the lockdown rules differed in every place, the punishments for breaking the rules were different, too. Many places around the world set up reporting lines. Those were phone numbers that people could call to report people who were breaking lockdown restrictions. That was one way police found out about those who were breaking restrictions.

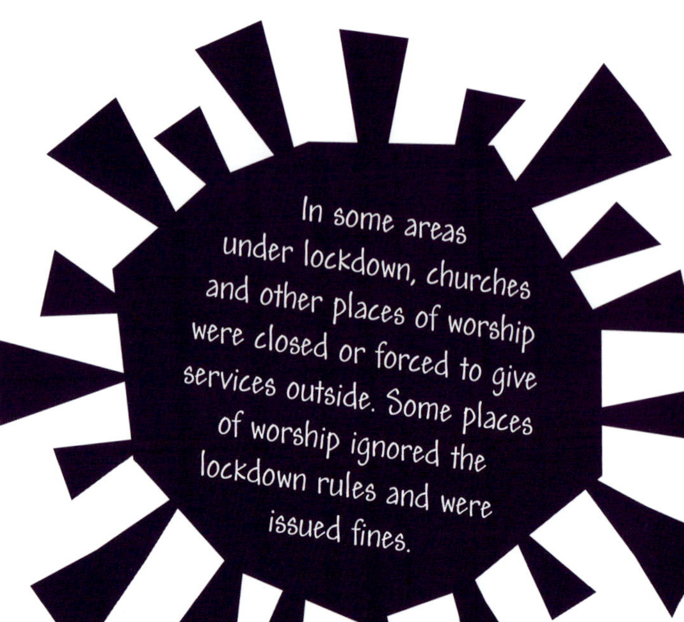

In some areas under lockdown, churches and other places of worship were closed or forced to give services outside. Some places of worship ignored the lockdown rules and were issued fines.

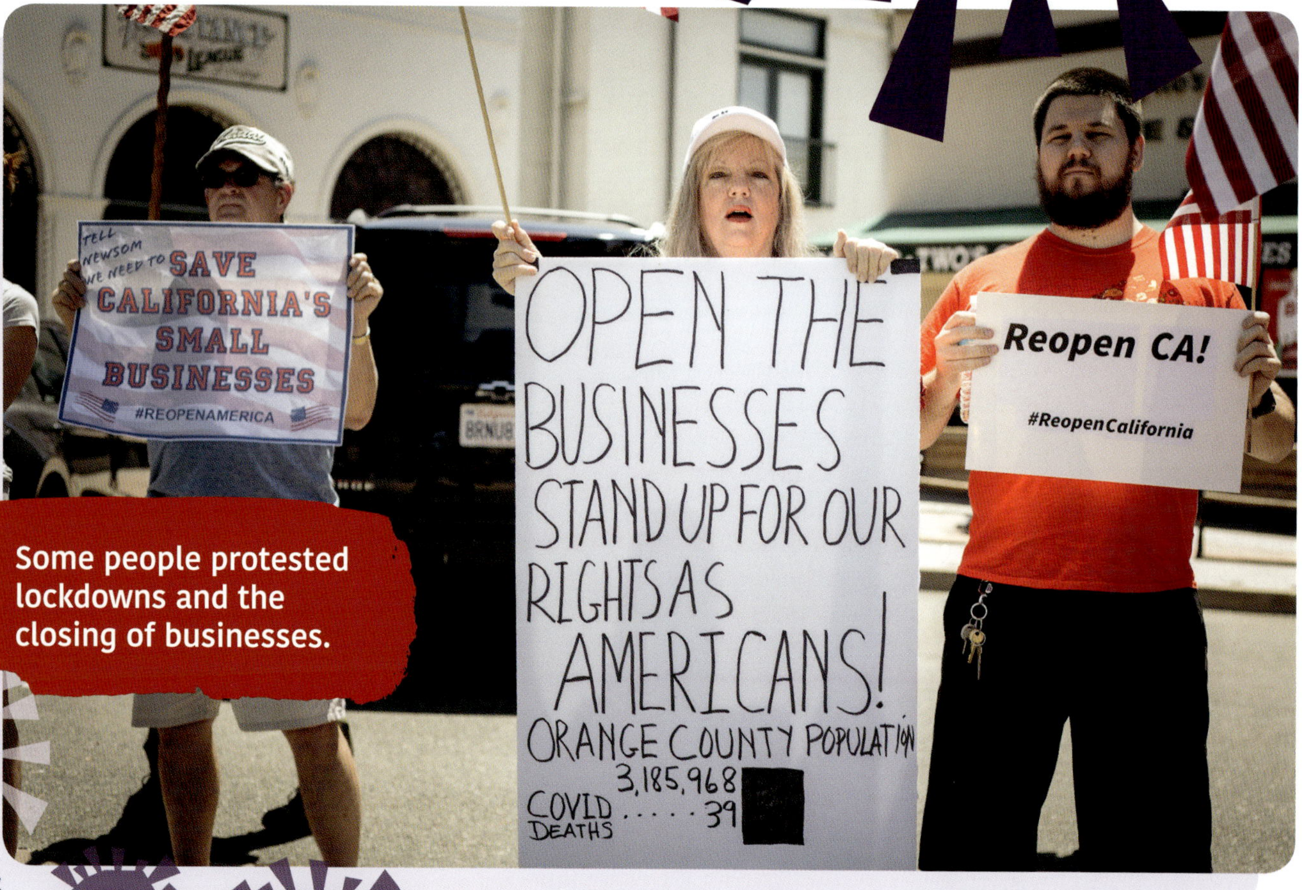

Some people protested lockdowns and the closing of businesses.

Facing Consequences

Australia was one country that imposed strict lockdowns in the early days of the pandemic. Those measures reduced cases quickly. Breaking the rules in Australia had serious consequences. Rule breakers could receive a $50,000 U.S. fine and up to 12 months in prison. Spain also fined more than one million people for breaking lockdown restrictions.

In Italy, people who tested positive for COVID-19 and broke their quarantine, going out in public, faced up to five years in prison. In South Africa, lockdown laws closed beaches during busy holiday seasons. Night time curfews were set from 9 p.m. to 6 a.m. Fines were set for breaking lockdown laws. These included one for "publishing any statement to deceive any other person about the infection status of any person." That carried a fine of 3,000 Rand ($197 U.S.). Leaving home during curfew carried a fine of 500 Rand ($33 U.S.). The measures were intended to keep people from gathering and spreading the virus, but also to deal with rumors and **misinformation** about the virus not being serious.

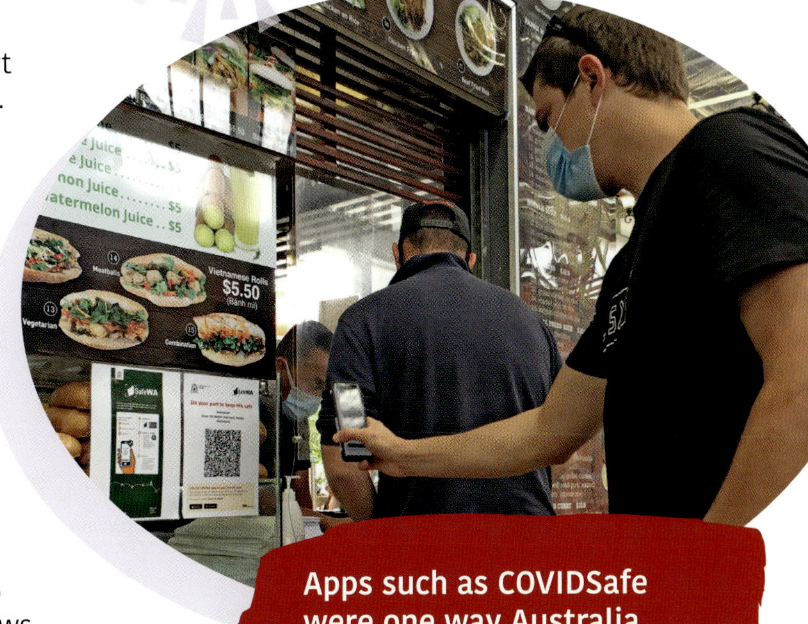

Apps such as COVIDSafe were one way Australia tracked people and located them if there was a positive case near them. They helped with testing people and identifying which areas were COVID-19 "hot spots," or areas with many cases.

PANDEMIC HERO

Vaccine Hunters Canada

When COVID-19 vaccines became more widely available in 2021, it quickly became apparent that some countries had well-organized rollout plans, and some did not. Canada's vaccine rollouts were managed by the country's 10 provinces and 3 territories. Many people were confused about how, where, and when to get their vaccinations. Some vaccines were offered at community clinics through provincial booking websites. Others were offered at drug stores, and some at temporary pop-up clinics. Vaccine Hunters Canada (VHC) came in to help people find locations where vaccines were available. The all-volunteer team of computer industry workers, social media workers, and others decided to put their skills to use. VHC set up a Twitter account and other social media. The group let Canadians know where vaccines were available, how many, and how to get them—in real time. Canada's largest city, Toronto, even partnered with the group to help get more people vaccinated.

Lockdown Lessons Learned

Lockdowns weren't meant to last forever. They were a disaster response measure brought in to control the spread of the virus by changing the actions of its hosts: humans.

Once the number of COVID-19 cases got under control, the plan was to carefully reopen businesses and allow people to gather. It was important to keep a close eye on the number of cases and hospitalizations as restrictions eased. Changes could then be made based on new information. Scientists were continually learning about the virus. It wasn't until July 2020 that the World Health Organization released research that proved the virus was airborne, and could linger in the air in crowded spaces. That was five months after the first lockdowns began. The research showed lockdowns were important measures for containing the virus. It also pointed out how some indoor spaces that could not be locked down needed better ways to keep people safe.

The lessons learned from lockdowns are both scientific and social. They can be used to develop better responses and planning for future pandemics and disasters.

Food factories were essential services. They remained open during lockdowns because they were needed to produce food for people. Factories have strict hygiene, but social distancing for workers can be difficult because of space.

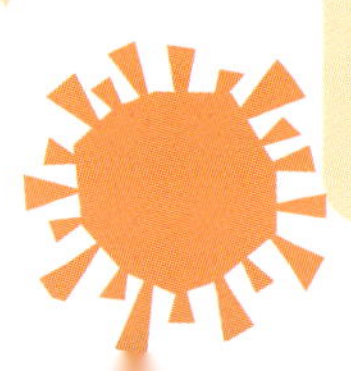

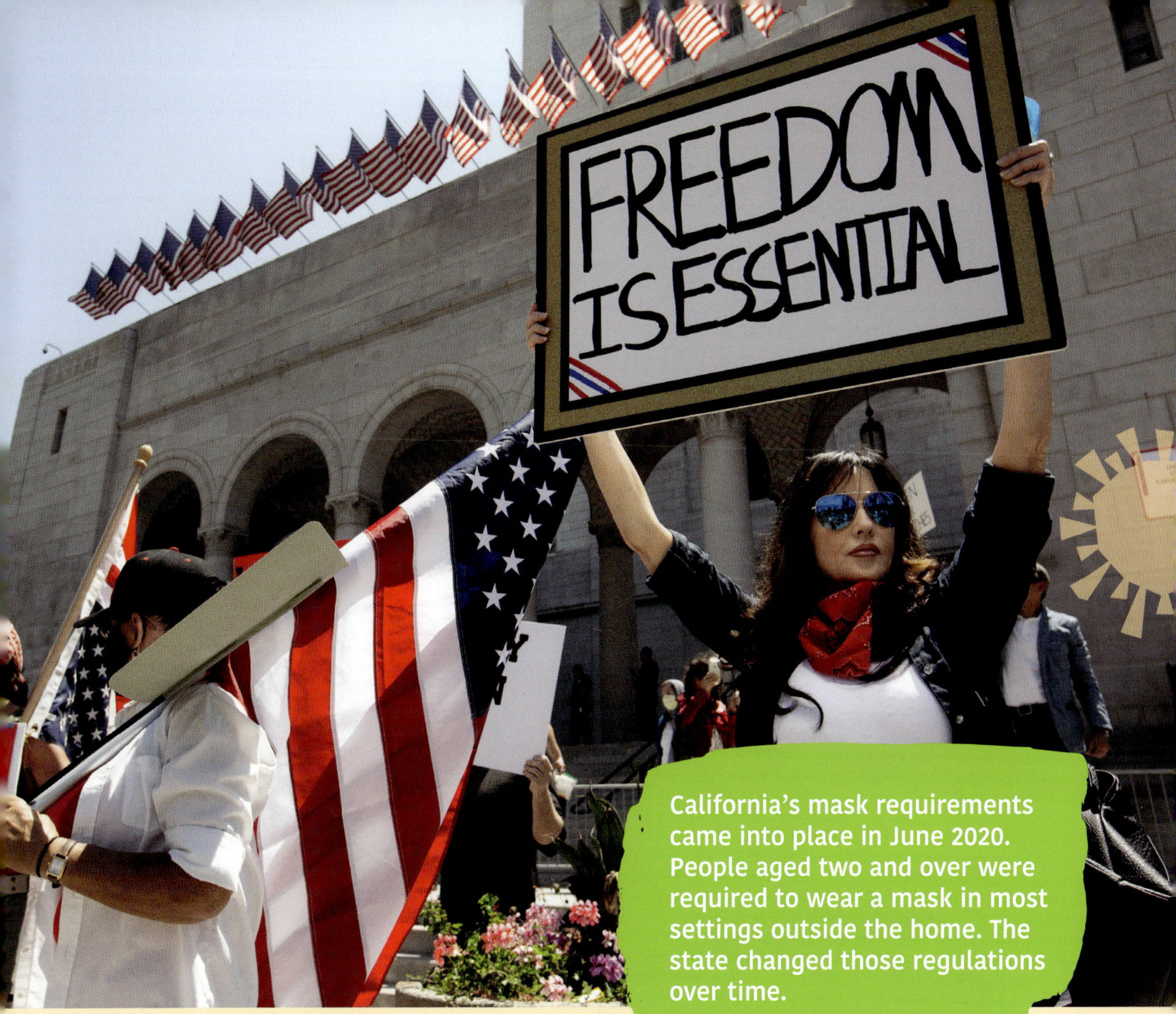

California's mask requirements came into place in June 2020. People aged two and over were required to wear a mask in most settings outside the home. The state changed those regulations over time.

What Lockdowns Meant

A year after the first lockdowns, governments and people around the world had learned many things. One was that keeping people safe and protecting health care systems required people to give up some of their freedoms. To slow the spread of a virus, people needed to limit their contact with others. However, not everyone was willing to make that sacrifice. Some people refused to wear masks and claimed the virus was not harmful. Others believed lockdowns were a way for governments to take more control of people's lives. Some protested the loss of personal freedoms.

Freedom vs Common Good

Democratic governments wrestled with the idea of limiting freedoms in lockdown. They didn't want to use power to control people's behaviors or take away **rights**—except when it threatened to cause harm to others. In a democracy, that is called the "harm principle." The risk of spreading COVID-19 was considered a threat of harm. During COVID-19, 17 American states required people who were not fully vaccinated to wear masks in most indoor settings. Most of Canada had mask regulations for all or part of the pandemic. Children and people with disabilities and medical conditions were exceptions.

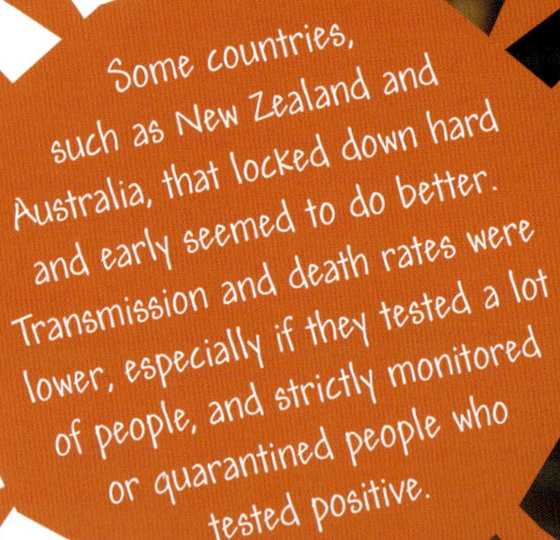

Some countries, such as New Zealand and Australia, that locked down hard and early seemed to do better. Transmission and death rates were lower, especially if they tested a lot of people, and strictly monitored or quarantined people who tested positive.

LONDON IS AT HIGH COVID ALERT LEVEL
Don't mix indoors with anyone you don't live with.
Hands
Face
Space

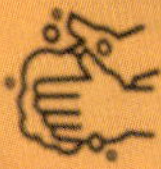

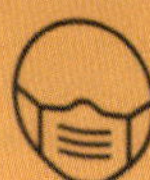

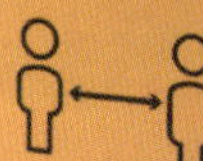

Some areas and countries, such as Canada and the United Kingdom, used rolling lockdowns and **tiered** levels of restrictions. Those lowered transmission rates for a while, but the rates increased when the restrictions ended. The tiered lockdowns were an attempt to save businesses and jobs, as well as lives.

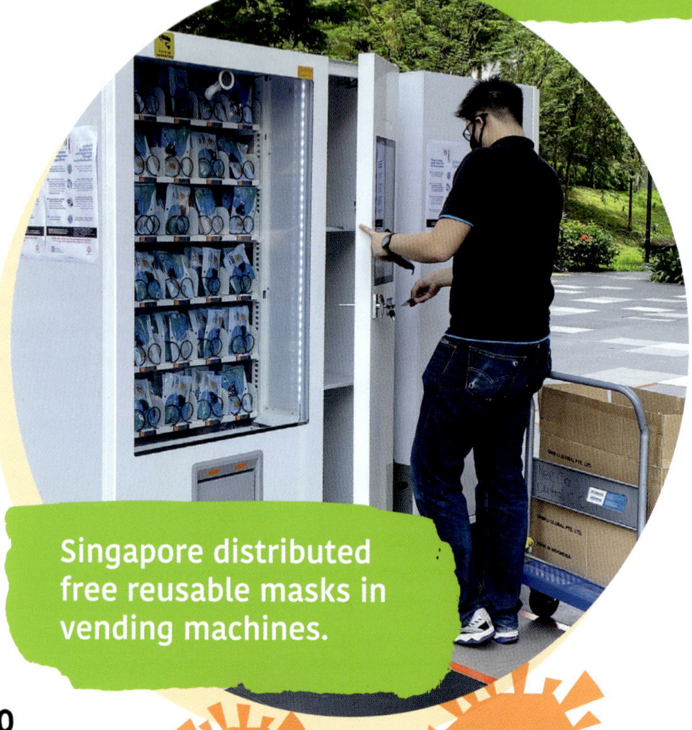

Singapore distributed free reusable masks in vending machines.

Learning to Cope

During the first wave, governments and citizens were learning how to deal with the first major pandemic in more than 100 years. New information about the disease came out daily. Public health guidelines and pandemic restrictions such as lockdowns were new measures that adapted to real-time situations. After the first wave, governments loosened lockdowns to help businesses recover. The number of people allowed to gather slowly increased. But the virus was still out there. As transmissions increased, many areas moved into a "second wave" of the pandemic. In many cases, lockdowns had to be reintroduced. Some countries had three and four waves when the virus spread to more people.

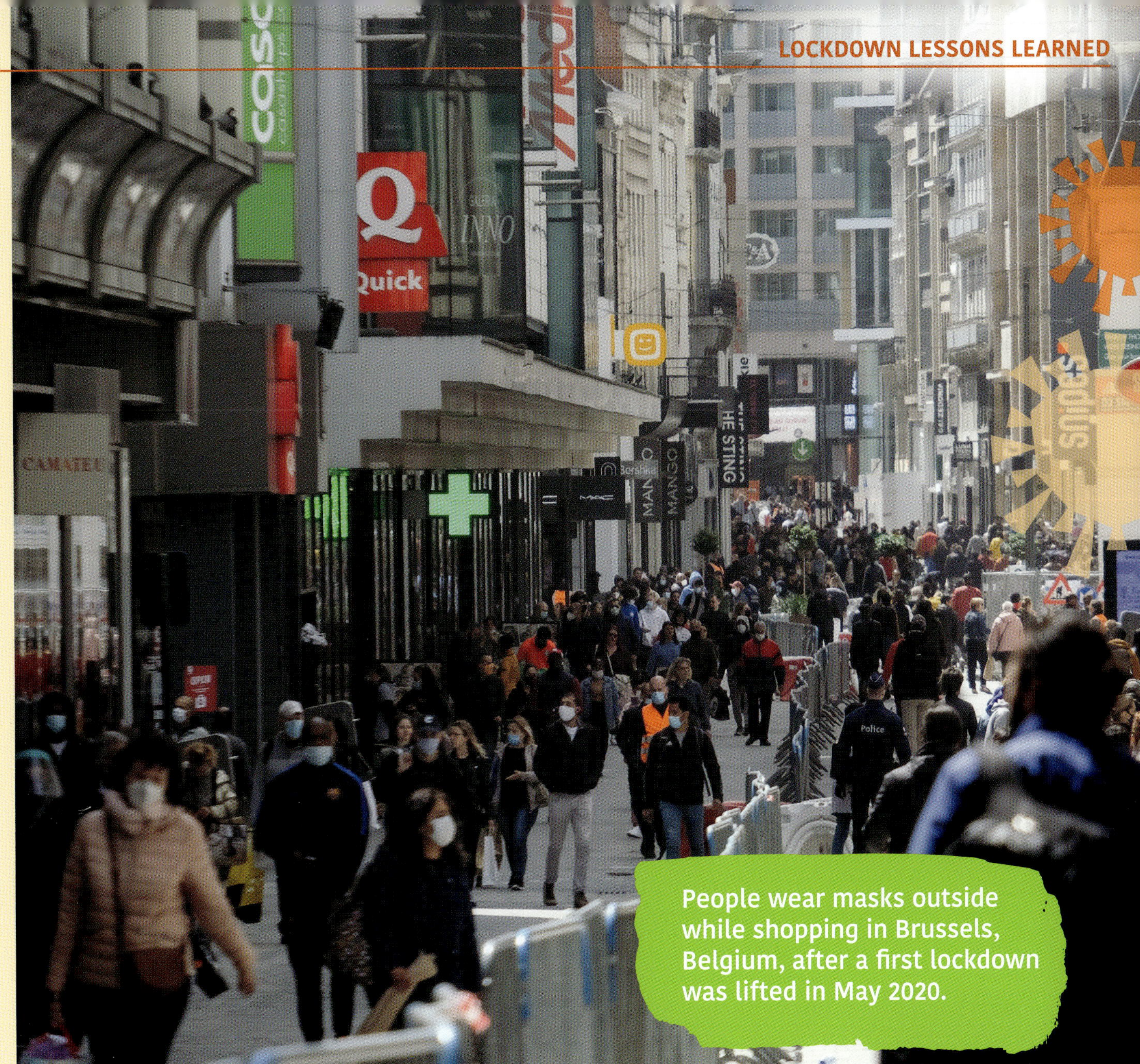

People wear masks outside while shopping in Brussels, Belgium, after a first lockdown was lifted in May 2020.

Lockdown Levels

Lockdown restrictions are beginning to loosen as the number of cases go down. But life has not gone back to normal just yet. Even in vaccinated populations, variants of the virus could create new waves of infection. Some countries and regions were hit harder by the virus than others. That was often related to population levels and **demographics**. In other words, it was related to the number of people who lived in an area, as well as how they lived and worked.

Some people worked in jobs that put them at high risk of getting the virus. Some lived in housing with many people, and could not isolate in their own homes if they contracted the virus. That made it more likely that their entire household would get COVID-19. As the pandemic wore on, it was easier to see that the types of lockdown methods played a big part in transmission rates. People who study government believe studying the many COVID-19 strategies will help make more effective plans for future disasters.

COVID-19 Changes

Living in lockdown was hard. People were isolated from their friends and family. Business closures cost people their jobs, making it difficult to pay their bills.

At the same time, lockdowns taught the world many lessons. Many businesses learned that their employees could be just as effective working from home as they were going in to the office. That led some business owners to close their physical office spaces permanently and allow their staff to work from wherever they chose. That changed the way people lived. Many who were living in small spaces in large cities decided to move. They didn't need to live close to work anymore. So some left bigger cities in favor of more space and a lower cost of living in smaller cities or more rural areas.

Separation and Resilience

Separated from their families, some people started learning new technologies that allowed them to communicate virtually. Grandparents became video-conferencing experts, relying on video calls to watch their grandchildren grow up. People turned to exercise, takeout food, and streaming services to cope with long stretches of loneliness and boredom.

Going out for supplies had to be pre-planned. Many things that people took for granted were no longer available or were in short supply.

COVID-19 showed what types of services and jobs were essential in an emergency situation. Those included health care workers, grocery store workers, factory workers, and delivery people.

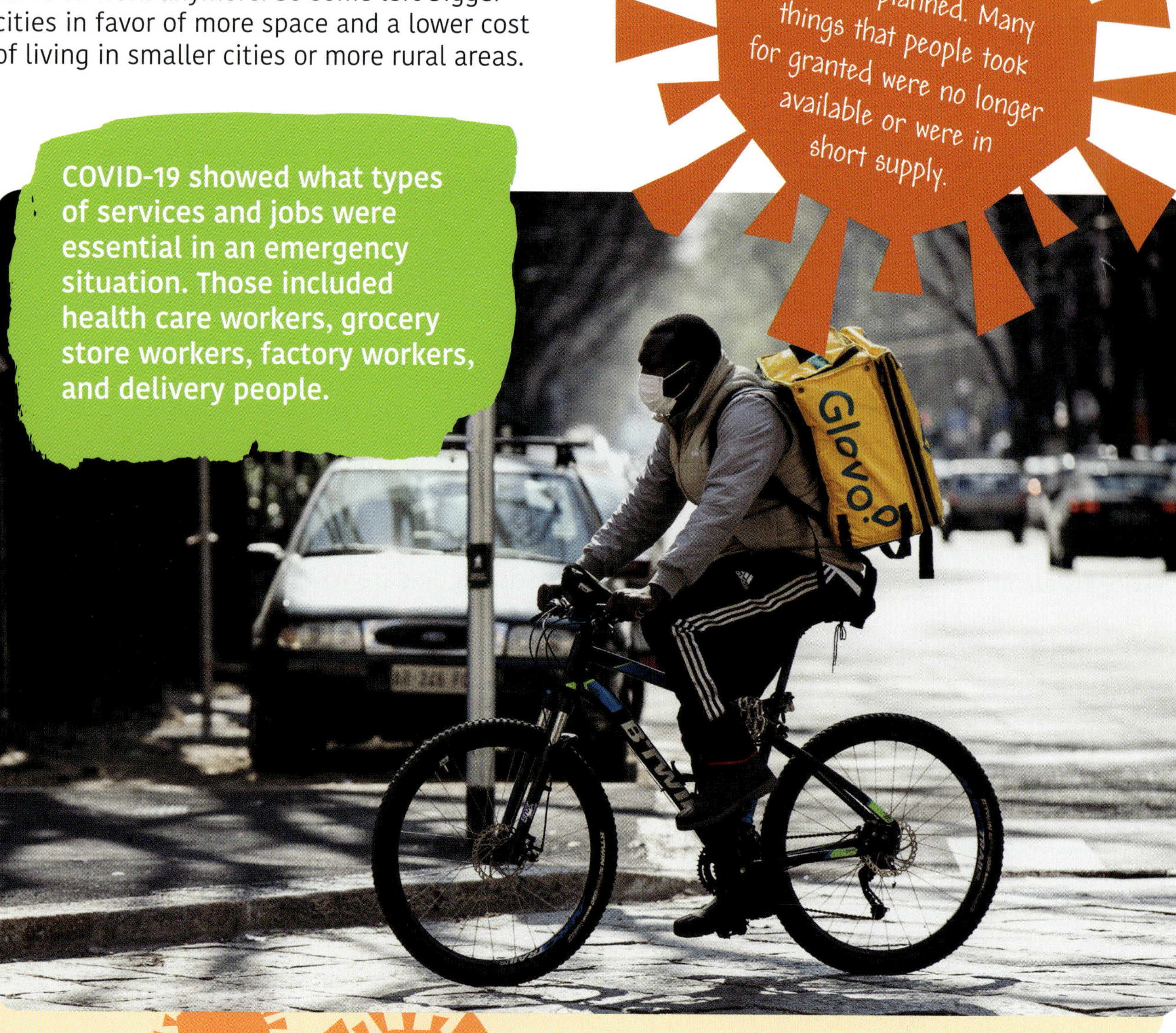

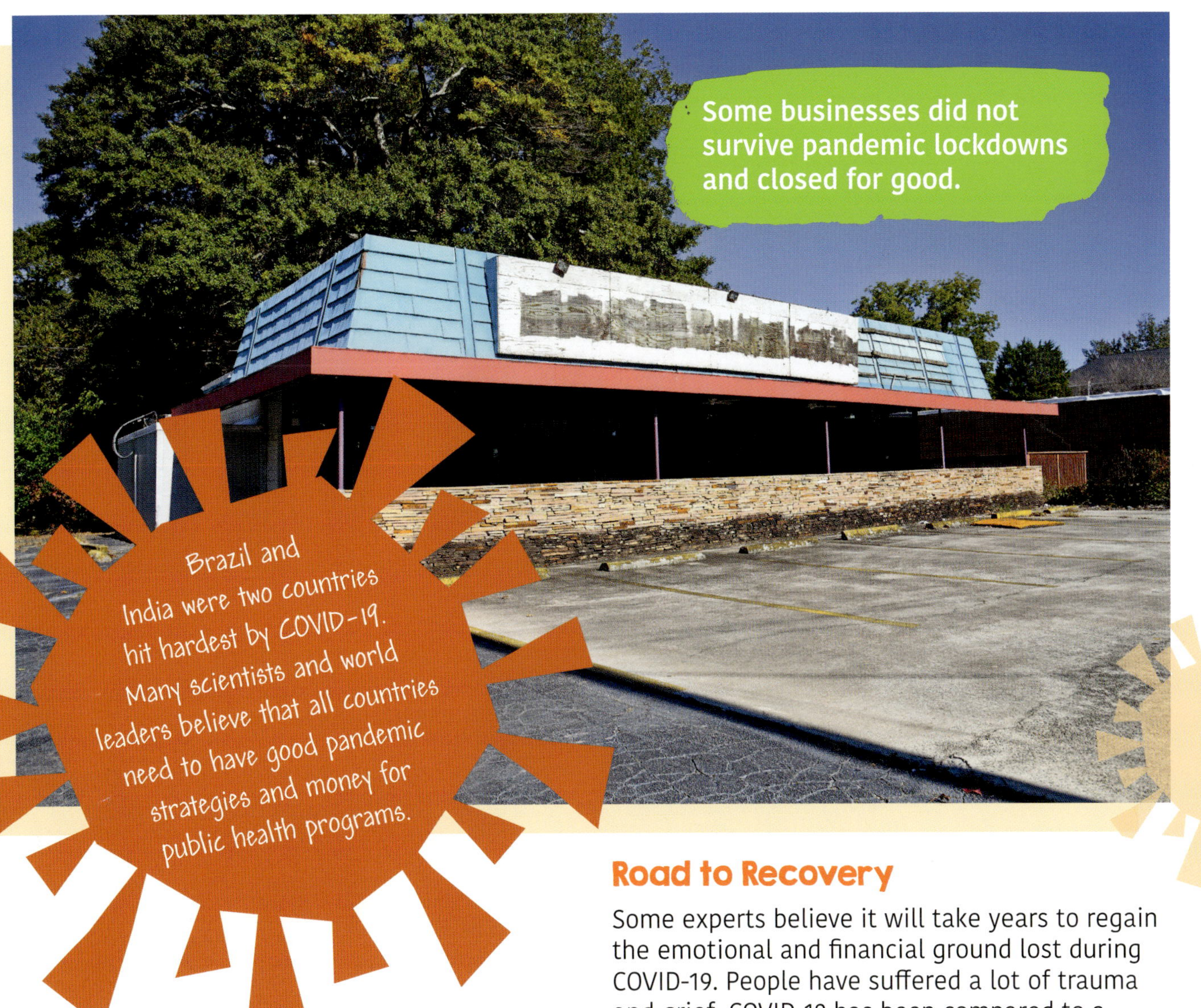

Some businesses did not survive pandemic lockdowns and closed for good.

Brazil and India were two countries hit hardest by COVID-19. Many scientists and world leaders believe that all countries need to have good pandemic strategies and money for public health programs.

Pandemic Inequalities

Lockdowns also highlighted the **inequalities** in society. While many people around the world lost their jobs, only some in wealthier countries could rely on government assistance to help pay their bills. Even then, it wasn't enough. Some people relied on friends, family, and donations to buy groceries and pay their bills. Others who were luckier built up savings because they could not spend their money on traveling, going out for fun, and eating at restaurants. The pandemic showed that some governments could afford to support people in need. It also showed how some countries needed support from other countries to vaccinate their populations.

Road to Recovery

Some experts believe it will take years to regain the emotional and financial ground lost during COVID-19. People have suffered a lot of trauma and grief. COVID-19 has been compared to a major war, such as **World War II**. That war left lasting scars on people and countries. But more Americans died from COVID-19 than the number of American soldiers who died during World War II. Economists point out that World War II also kick-started years of economic growth.

In May 2021, the U.S. government released a $6 trillion dollar budget plan designed to fire up the country's economy and create jobs. During COVID-19, governments saw how important science and scientific research was in saving lives and creating treatments and vaccines. Some have pledged to invest more in scientific research. It is likely there will be other pandemics in the future, so pandemic planning will also be needed.

Bibliography

Intro

Feng, Emily. "Wuhan's Lockdown Memories 1 Year Later: Pride, Anger, Deep Pain." NPR, January 23, 2021. https://www.npr.org/sections/goatsandsoda/2021/01/23/959618838/wuhans-lockdown-memories-one-year-later-pride-anger-deep-pain

Chapter 1

Jegelevicius, Linas. "Belarus and coronavirus: Lukashenko's business-as-usual approach is 'mind-blowing negligence." EuroNews, April 21, 2020. https://bit.ly/2MBUDtm

Sanche, Steven, Yen Ting Lin, Chonggang Xu, et al. "High Contagiousness and Rapid Spread of Severe Acute Respiratory Syndrome Coronavirus 2." Centers for Disease Control and Prevention, July 2020. https://wwwnc.cdc.gov/eid/article/26/7/20-0282_article

Sandford, Alasdair. "Coronavirus: Half of humanity now on lockdown as 90 countries call for confinement. EuroNews, April 23, 2020. https://bit.ly/3r0JoJZ

Sudworth, John. "Coronavirus: Wuhan emerges from the harshest of lockdowns." BBC News, April 8, 2020. https://bbc.in/3ktVtoe

Chapter 2

McDonough, Annie. "Remote learning challenges will likely continue in New York." City & State New York, August 30, 2020. https://bit.ly/3swWpel

"Online shopping has doubled during the pandemic, Statistics Canada says." CBC News, July 24, 2020. https://www.cbc.ca/news/business/online-shopping-covid-19-1.5661818

"Online shopping sales surge by 99% in Canada amid coronavirus pandemic." Global News, July 24, 2020. https://globalnews.ca/news/7213764/coronavirus-online-shopping-canada/

Chapter 3

C "Economic Impact Reports," World Travel & Tourism Council. https://wttc.org/Research/Economic-Impact

Hall, Stefan. "This is how COVID-19 is affecting the music industry." World Economic Forum, May 27, 2020. https://www.weforum.org/agenda/2020/05/this-is-how-covid-19-isaffecting-the-music-industry/

Kochhar, Rakesh. "Unemployment rose higher in three months of COVID-19 than it did in two years of the Great Recession." Pew Research Center, June 11, 2020. https://pewrsr.ch/3q0Zwtw

Melimopoulos, Elizabeth. "What's driving the COVID lockdown protests?" Al Jazeera, February 7, 2021. https://bit.ly/3q1Bgas

Panchal, Nirmita, Rabah Kamal, Cynthia Cox, and Rachel Garfield. "The Implications of COVID-19 for Mental Health and Substance Use." Kaiser Family Foundation, February 10, 2021. https://bit.ly/3pZUuxr

Patton, Mike. "Pre And Post Coronavirus Unemployment Rates By State, Industry, Age Group, And Race." Forbes, June 28, 2020. https://bit.ly/3kwlfrX

Press, Benjamin, and Thomas Carothers. "Worldwide Protests in 2020: A Year in Review." Carnegie Endowment for International Peace, December 21, 2020. https://carnegieendowment.org/2020/12/21/worldwide-protests-in-2020-year-in-review-pub-83445

Richardson, Lisa, and Allison Crawford. "How Indigenous Communities in Canada Organized an Exemplary Public Health Response to COVID." Scientific American, October 27, 2020. https://www.scientificamerican.com/article/how-indigenouscommunities-in-canada-organized-an-exemplary-public-healthresponse-to-covid/

Singh, Shweta, Deblina Roy, Krittika Sinha, et al. "Impact of COVID-19 and lockdown on mental health of children and adolescents: A narrative review with recommendations." Psychiatry Research, August 24, 2020. https://www.ncbi.nlm.nih.gov/pmc/articles/PMC7444649/

Slotnick, David. "COVID-19 could eliminate 197 million travel industry jobs and wipe $5.5 trillion from the global GDP, a trade group warns."Business Insider, August 17, 2020. https://bit.ly/37SwjL7

"The retail evolution's great acceleration: How to maneuver in the pandemic-driven recession." Deloitte. https://bit.ly/3bHyqCI

Chapter 4

Morgan, Sarah Blake. "At funerals in virus outbreak, mourning is from a distance." ABC News, April 4, 2020. https://abcn.ws/3uG9295

"New fines for breaking South Africa's lockdown laws – what you will pay." BusinessTech, May 8, 2020. https://bit.ly/3sxckt7

Paperny, Anna, and Moira Warburton. "Canadians seeking vaccines rely on web-savvy volunteers." Reuters, May 6, 2021. https://www.reuters.com/world/americas/canadians-seekingvaccines-rely-web-savvy-volunteers-2021-05-06/

Ward, Alex. "How coronavirus is changing the ways we grieve and mourn the dead." Vox, April 7, 2020. https://bit.ly/3aYe096

Chapter 5

"Biden unveils 'once in a generation' spending plan." BBC News, April 1, 2021. https://www.bbc.com/news/business-56594349

Haltiwanger, John. "More Americans have now died from COVID-19 than the number of US troops killed during World War II." Business Insider, January 20, 2021. https://www.businessinsider.com/more-americans-dead-covid-19-usbattle-deaths-wwii-2020-12

McLaughlin, Eliott C. "10 lessons learned in a year of COVID-19 lockdown." CNN, March 13, 2021. https://www.cnn.com/2021/03/13/us/lockdown-lessons-learnedcovid-19/index.html

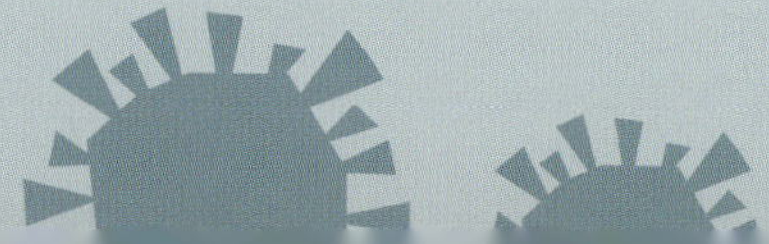

Timeline

December 10, 2019 One of the first suspected coronavirus patients falls ill in Wuhan, China.

December 30, 2019 Wuhan doctor, Li Wenliang, shares information about the new virus online.

December 31, 2019 Chinese authorities alert the World Health Organization (WHO) of an outbreak of pneumonia cases in Wuhan, China.

January 20, 2020 CDC announces that three American airports will begin screening for the virus.

January 23, 2020 Wuhan, China is put into lockdown, but 5 million people leave the city without being screened for the illness.

January 31, 2020 China locks down.

February 2, 2020 Global air travel is restricted.

February 11, 2020 WHO announces that the novel coronavirus will be named COVID-19.

March 11, 2020 WHO declares COVID-19 a pandemic and calls for global response to contain it.

March 19, 2020 California issues statewide stay-at-home order.

April 4, 2020 More than 1 million cases are confirmed worldwide.

June 8, 2020 New Zealand lifts all lockdown restrictions and declares itself virus-free.

August 8, 2020 U.S. surpasses 5 million cases.

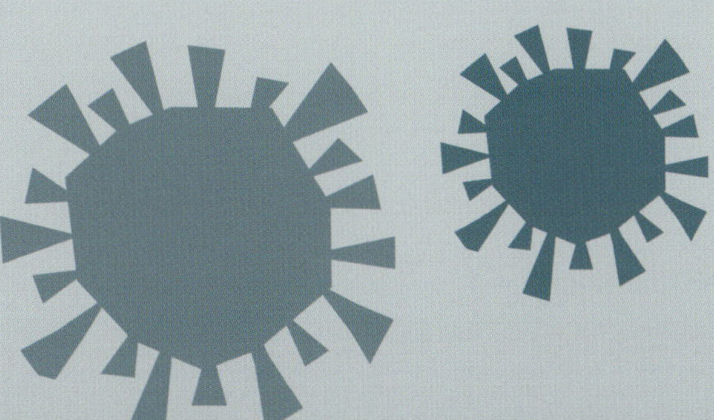

November 9, 2020 Pfizer and BioNTech announce that their vaccine candidate is more than 90 percent effective in preventing COVID-19.

December 26, 2020 Global cases surpass 80 million.

December 30, 2020 Ireland reverts to full lockdown.

January 5, 2021 The world surpasses two million COVID-19 deaths.

May 28, 2021 Melbourne, Australia enters a seven-day lockdown—the city's fifth lockdown.

June 1, 2021 U.K. announces zero daily COVID-19 deaths.

June 2, 2021 World COVID-19 rates rise again as virus variants spread. Vaccines prove effective in preventing serious disease and deaths as world death total surpasses 4 million.

July 12, 2021 The WHO says more equitable, or equal access to vaccines is key to controlling COVID-19 throughout the world.

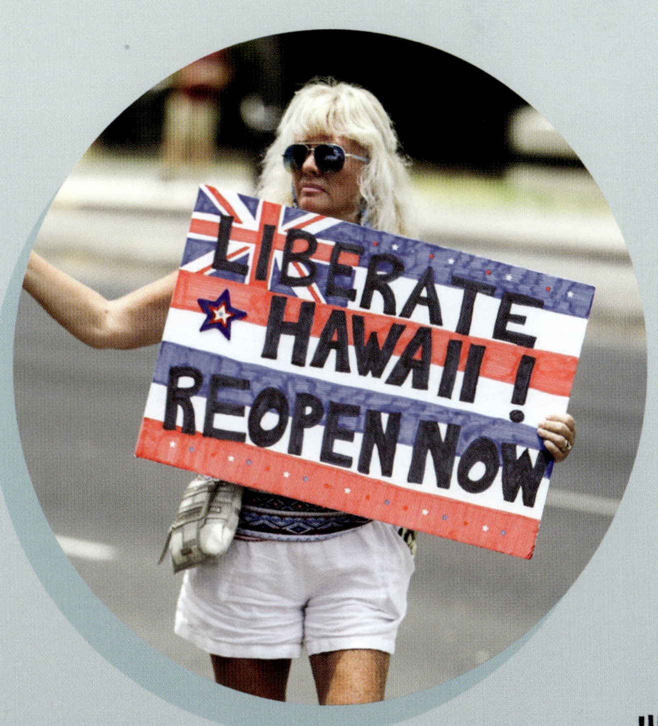

Learning More

Books

LaBonte, Lisa. *Resilient Youth: Emotional Wellbeing in the Wake of the COVID-19 Global Pandemic.* Van Wagenen Publishing, 2020.

O'Brien, Cynthia. *Wars Waged Under the Microscope: COVID-19.* Crabtree Publishing, 2021.

Hustad, Douglas. Understanding COVID-19. Core Library, 2020.

Websites

Watch and read stories about how teens across the U.S. adapted to lockdowns and faced changes during the pandemic.
https://www.pbs.org/newshour/nation/how-teens-adapted-and-changed-during-the-pandemic

Youth group games that can be played over Skype or Zoom at times when you can't be with friends or family.
https://youthgroupgames.com.au/collection/virtual-youth-group-games/

This website has a number of free COVID-19 ebooks for kids
https://www.scjpp;,emta;jea;tj.prg/,edoa/SOM/Microsites/NCSMH/Documents/COCID-19/COVID=Bppls-Resources.-For-Children-final.pdf

Glossary

anxiety Feelings of worry and fear.

business models Designs for how a business will be run

Centers for Disease Control and Prevention (CDC) A branch of the United States Public Health Service that investigates and controls diseases

collaboration Working together on something

consumer A person who buys goods

contagiousness How easily a virus is passed between people

coronavirus A family of viruses that cause illnesses ranging from the common cold to COVID-19.

curfews Rules that require people to stay at home during certain hours

democratic Describes a system of government in which people elect their leaders

demographics Characteristics of a certain group or population, such as age, ethnicity, religion, income, and more

depression A mental illness or disorder in which a person feels persistent sadness,